MID-LIFE CRISES

MID·LIFE CRISES

by

William E. Hulme

THE WESTMINSTER PRESS

Philadelphia

Copyright © 1980 The Westminster Press

All rights reserved—no part of this book may be repro-
duced in any form without permission in writing from
the publisher, except by a reviewer who wishes to quote
brief passages in connection with a review in magazine
or newspaper.

Scripture quotations from the Revised Standard Ver-
sion of the Bible are copyrighted 1946, 1952, © 1971,
1973 by the Division of Christian Education of the
National Council of the Churches of Christ in the
U.S.A., and are used by permission.

Book Design by Dorothy Alden Smith

First edition

Published by The Westminster Press®
Philadelphia, Pennsylvania

PRINTED IN THE UNITED STATES OF AMERICA
9 8 7 6 5 4 3 2 1

Library of Congress Cataloging in Publication Data

Hulme, William Edward, 1920–
  Mid-life crises.

  (Christian care books ; 7)
  Bibliography: p.
  1. Middle age—Conduct of life.
2. Family—Religious life. I. Title.
II. Series.
BJ1690.H84   170′.2′022   80–11539
ISBN 0–664–24324–X

Contents

Foreword

I responded positively to the invitation to write this book because I know something about the subject from personal experience and as a result have something to say about it. I am writing primarily to Christian parents who are in mid-life, and who therefore may be experiencing some common concerns. Because as Christians we are *in* the world, but not *of* it, we experience a distinct tension in relating to the cultural values that press in upon us. Christian parents have a difficult task in rearing their children according to the Way of Christ, and assisting them at the same time to cope in some positive manner with the opposing ways that are all about us. The task is complicated by the fact that we parents to some extent have bought into these cultural values. This in turn contributes to mid-life crises, which are more culturally than biologically conditioned.

But such crises can be creative. Parents also have needs and are also in a growth process. Crises can facilitate this growth.

I am grateful to Wayne Oates for giving me the opportunity to write this book. It is not a subject I would have selected on my own. Once I began writing, however, I became aware of how relevant it is to most aspects of the Christian life. Truly, mid-life is a great time in one's pilgrimage. Unfortunately, because of our cultural focus on youth and young adulthood and our almost pathological fear of aging, this reality is not recognized. If this book can help those who are in this time of life to realize the potential of these years, I would feel all the better about my effort.

W.E.H.

St. Paul, Minnesota

1. Mid-Life Crisis—What Causes It? Who Has It?

George made an appointment with his minister, but he was not looking forward to the meeting. He knew why his wife had sought counsel with the pastor and why the pastor invited him to do likewise. He clenched his teeth as he entered the pastor's study—a symbol of his determination that nothing would deter him. "She's a good woman and a good mother," he said, "but I've got to do what I've got to do."

"You want a divorce," the pastor said, helping him to get to the point.

"Yes," he said. "I'm not satisfied—haven't been for the past several years. She's not interested in my interests. I've got to act now before it's too late."

"Your wife is aware of her past insensitivity, and she's willing to change," the pastor said.

"I know," said George, "but it's too late. No matter who gets hurt—my wife, my son, even my aged mother—I've got to seek my own fulfillment and I have to do it now."

What brings a man like George—a successful stockbroker and church worker—to such a desperate decision? There are, of course, many factors involved that are peculiar to

George. His nineteen-year-old son, rebellious all through his teens, is not fulfilling his father's expectations. The fact that George has reached mid-life in our contemporary American culture, however, also has something to do with it.

Marge represents a quite different case. She has arrived at an age that she considered old when her mother was that age, and she feels it. Her youngest child is in his first year at college. Two other children are married. Marge has always been sensitive, but of late supersensitive. Her children are annoyed because she has become increasingly demanding of them when they are involved in establishing their own lives. Her marriage with Roger has never developed much companionship. Now Roger is all there is left in a home once bustling with energetic children. Roger finds reasons to remain at work even more than before. Like the children, he smarts from Marge's accusations and demands.

Behind her crotchety and accusatory demeanor Marge is a frightened woman. Who desires a middle-aged woman whose only future is in growing older, becoming less needed —and, she fears, less wanted? In a moment of honesty with an old school friend, she acknowledged that she was depressed and doing a lot of unhealthy brooding about death.

Biological Factors Not Basic

I have described two persons who are in the midst of a severe mid-life crisis. If you are approaching mid-life or are in the midst of it, perhaps you have some concerns yourself. What, basically, is a mid-life crisis? What causes it? Do all middle-aged people go through it? If you are a woman, you have known for many years that you would go through menopause if you lived long enough. Biological changes would then occur which would make it impossible any longer for you to conceive and to bear a child. If you are a man, you may be aware of the talk these days about male menopause. Your father probably wasn't even aware of the term, although a few people in those days referred to a "male climacteric." Today there appears to be more emphasis on male than female menopause.

With women, biological factors are obviously involved in menopause. Some people have surmised that there is a more modified biological factor also in a male "change of life," but there is no clinical confirmation of this. Biological factors, however, are not the basic issue in a mid-life crisis. As one authority put it, hot flashes, not depression, go with female menopause. One's psychological response to the hot flashes, however, may precipitate a crisis. Despite the possibility of glandular changes also in men, the only concrete data regarding male mid-life crises are psychological or spiritual. One writer says there is no such thing as male menopause —only male mid-life crises, which she describes as a "psychological crossroads" that can be "turned to the positive" (Nancy Mayer).

What is the nature of the psychological crisis? Actually it is a crisis in one's outlook on life. It is spiritual in nature— a crisis in values. A good insight into this crisis is the view of it as a type of "neo-adolescence." Questions about the meaning of life that troubled you in adolescence may return in mid-life. We ask the inescapable questions about our identity, our vocation, our purpose for living. In adolescence we become intensely aware of our individuality, our aloneness, as we begin to lose our childhood attachments to our family. It can be a frightening experience.

This same sense of aloneness may return in mid-life and it can be just as frightening. In adolescence we felt the guilt of our *fallenness* as fantasies and feelings beyond our control seemed to corrupt us. In mid-life we may experience a recurrent sense of this self-judgment—even self-hatred. In the same family, adolescent children and their middle-aged parents may be going through the same sort of anguish over their identity.

One factor that may precipitate a mid-life crisis is the change in our relationship to our children. Our limits as parents, which we were aware of even when the children were small, may now seem overwhelming. The dreams we had for our children may turn into fears as we see them influenced by the fluctuating mood of the times. Old props and trusted formulas that we had counted on heretofore may no longer seem dependable. We whom society holds responsible for our children seem in reality to have so little influence upon them. As younger parents we may have asserted what we would or would not tolerate from your children. When one of these nontolerable situations later arises, our power to prevent it seems to dissipate.

What power we may still retain with our older children needs to be used wisely. Parents of teenagers, says a psychiatrist, need to resist these children when they show disrespect for the values they have been taught. But then he qualifies that resistance. "Too much resistance blocks progress," he says, "and too little allows change without regard to consequences." How much is "too much" and how little is "too little"? These are the questions that frustrate parents. Besides, who would have thought that our children would ever seriously question our values or our religion?

CHANGE IN VOCATIONAL GOALS

Another factor that may be involved in mid-life crises is the vocational goals one has had in the first half of life. How have you measured worth, value, success, failure? If you are a professional person, you may have bought into the value system of the professional world by which you evaluate your worth. As a parent or a spouse, by what standards do you determine whether you are a good mother or father, a good wife or husband? Mid-life can be a difficult time when you are not faring well by whatever standards you may be using to evaluate yourself. Because we can see more clearly the limits that lie ahead, we are vulnerable in mid-life to doubts about whether or not we are "making it."

Until recently, perhaps you were able to put off some basic questions about the meaning and purpose of life. If you were "doing well" in the business world or as a parent, this was sufficient encouragement to keep you going. In the latter half of life, however, it may be more difficult to devote your energies toward your old pursuits. We can see why alcohol and drugs appeal as diversions from the uneasiness we may experience within ourselves. An extramarital affair offers the same attraction.

Those who succumb to these distractions usually rationalize their motives. It's the pressure of business, or the lack of support at home, or the need for companionship. Rarely would one explain one's actions by saying, "I am running from the prospect of aging, or dying, or from the specter of my failure as a person." In mid-life we have moved beyond utilizing our energies to establish ourselves in the adult world. Our goals in the second half of life may not be nearly so concrete as before. The exception may be the woman who is now moving out from a life that was dedicated to home-making into a new career in the world. People in mid-life need something new to "grab" them and a new career can do that.

The comparison of mid-life crises to the crises of adolescence needs qualifying. Our bodies are older. We no longer have the physical energy of our youth. We may have put on weight, our joints may be less limber, our organs less robust, and our blood pressure too high. Some physical deterioration may result from past sins against our bodies—too little exercise, too much sugar, fat, or starch in our diets, and too much stress.

These physical deteriorations force us into a change of life-style. Jess Lair, popular writer on quality living, accredits a heart attack with changing his life-style. Paul Brenner, a popular lecturer and professor of medicine in the San Diego area, hurt his knee while jogging. Sidelined by surgery, Brenner reevaluated his life and decided to quit the practice of medicine. Declaring that he had paid his debt to medicine, he chose to devote the latter half of his life to doing the things he really wanted to do. Reflecting on his experience, he poses the question, Do you need a heart attack or cancer to "make today count"?

Our bodies are a convenient place to deposit our inner tensions—including those associated with mid-life. While the idea of psychosomatic illness has been around a long time, our awareness of the psychological input into our somatic pains continues to expand. We no longer divide illnesses into organic and psychosomatic; rather, we delineate only the degree of psychosomatic input. Our body is the culturally accepted location into which to displace our anxieties and depressions.

Though often bypassed by excursions into alcohol or illicit sex, or displaced into bodily pains, gnawing questions about the end of life come to the fore in middle age. Where is it all leading? What is it all about? What values do we need for facing the end of fertility, the end of work, the end of life? Death is a stark threat in adolescence. In young adulthood it is more easily diverted by illusions of immortality. The beginning of marriage, the starting of a family, establishing oneself in the world, tend to obscure one's awareness of endings. At the halfway mark it is more difficult to sustain such illusions. "April is full"—as the song goes—but "November is hollow." Our own parents, who seemed so immortal to us as children, are now growing old. How long, we wonder, will they be able to live alone? How long before we will be where they are?

Like adolescence, mid-life is a time for change. Any period in which ultimate questions come to the fore is potentially a period of growth. But growth can be painful. No wonder we are tempted to take the detour into pain relievers of all kinds.

The Christian Family and the World

I have been describing a crisis that is common to people in our culture. Does this description apply to Christians as well—in particular to Christian families? The Christian

family, despite its distinctiveness, shares the common life of
people in this world. As Jesus said, Christians are *in* the
world. We are susceptible to all human diseases. We are not
spared because of our faith from the problems, crises, and
even tragedies that afflict other families in our society. We
used to say that the drug problem with youth could not
occur in Christian families. Such assurances are now exposed as wishful thinking. Christian families have experienced all the modern afflictions—youth on drugs, alcoholism, sexual indiscretions, babies born out of wedlock,
legal offense and incarceration, mental illness and suicide.
Sociological factors beyond the family influence family
members. Our society has been undergoing a change in
what previously were accepted values and priorities. Your
teenage children are not being reared in the same social
environment you were. Your parents had child-rearing problems also, but not to the extent that you as parents are
experiencing.

The same social changes that affect our parental roles also
affect our marriages. One might have received the impression from wedding homilies of the past that marital harmony was the natural outcome of Christian commitment.
Today we observe an increasing amount of marital dishar-
mony not only in the world but also among Christians.
There is a decided increase of divorce among church people,
including even the clergy. Few of us have not had close
friends who have gone through divorce. The frustrations of
mid-life are easily projected into the marriage relationship.
Instead of dealing directly with frustrations over aging or
self-worth, we divert them and they reappear in marital
conflicts. George, with whom we began this chapter, is a

case in point. In a previous day he would have stayed with his wife even though he was dissatisfied. In our day he is likely to leave her in the search of an illusory fulfillment— a modern-day euphemism for the fountain of youth.

There is also a positive side to social change. Old pressures to present a good front regardless of how bad the situation are removed. Families then are freed to admit their troubles and seek the help they need. Because so many family problems are coming to light, more ways and better means have been developed for coping with them. When old pressures to conform are removed, we have more options. This may mean more ways to run from our problems. Or if we decide not to run, we may be ready to come to grips with our problems.

Not of the World

The Christian family, though in the world, is also "not of the world." It has resources from a realm beyond. These resources are often kept in reserve—something like an extra savings account for a "rainy day." If we find ourselves called upon to use them, we know things are really bad. We turn to our religious resources in times of crises. Otherwise we depend on our own resources. So long as we feel in control of our lives, we are *in* the world and *of* the world. When our control breaks down, we turn to another realm for help.

Mid-life crises may be precipitated by this sort of double-mindedness, for the confidence that depends on our being "on top of things" can be shaken in mid-life. The very fact that we are aging, that our lives are half over, is beyond our control. We may have preferred to "walk by sight" rather than "by faith." What happens then when what we see is no longer reassuring?

Our children may take our teaching of the Christian way more seriously than we do. In their innocence they may not suspect our double-mindedness. Later in adolescence when they do perceive it, they may become quite critical of our "hypocrisy." Because they may take their faith more seriously, our children may have more conflicts with the world than we have. They are less likely to compromise with injustice, less willing to adjust to the status quo, less likely to share our prejudices, since they are not so heavily invested in the world. For this reason, they may experience the *cross* more than their parents. The social ostracism which some young people endure simply because they refuse to go along with their peers causes a good deal of suffering. They are, in effect, taking up their cross. It is a high price to pay for being in the world but not of it. I have learned much from my children about what it means to be Christian. I can be swept along by the status quo and by conformity to cultural compromises—even in the church—until one of my children raises the unwelcome question, Is it really the Way of Christ? For whatever corruption I may have escaped by not compromising with the world—and I am never sure just how much this is—I am indebted in great part to my family.

How can we—parents and children—be in the world and yet not be of the world? Obviously it isn't easy. We are tempted to withdraw from the world, which is really impossible, or to compromise with it, which is quite possible. In mid-life we may raise the question, along with our teenagers, about these compromises. Our confrontation with life's limits may move us anew to ask what it means to be in but not of the world. The question leads us to resources beyond our own.

A Potentially Creative Conflict

The mid-life crisis can be creative—a conflict that generates a whole new outlook on life. We human beings are predisposed to inertia. Unless we are highly stimulated, we tend to stay as we are. Fortunately life is not disposed to support inertia. As Gail Sheehy has illustrated in her book *Passages*, we experience many passages throughout our lives, not simply at adolescence and mid-life, although these are of primary importance. We move from one orientation to life to another and the passage is usually marked by anxiety. Why, then, if passages are painful, do we experience them? Because human life is a moving, dynamic process! God created us with an inherent need to *grow*. We change with our years and what satisfied us before may not satisfy us now. This is the counterforce to our inertia—an indigenous stimulation for growth.

Though we are predisposed to experience conflict between our inertia and our need to grow, we are not predisposed to resolve the conflict creatively. Sheehy's stories of people in passages and our own observations reveal tragic as well as inspiring consequences of these conflicts. Some of us seem to get stymied in the passage. Although dissatisfied with our old ways, we lack the courage to enter into new ways. So we stagnate and use our energies destructively to make ourselves and our families miserable.

God has not called us to such a waste of our potential. Rather, we are called to be responsible, so that our conflicts and crises may be the means for new life and growth. Some of us need a push from the outside—an illness, a loss of job, a family crisis—before we are ready to move. Sometimes this push may come from something less drastic, such as a caring confrontation by a good friend or a concerned group.

Your family—as marvelous as it is—needs an extended family. This may be one of the resources you also need in mid-life crisis. Children need adults in addition to their parents with whom to relate. Parents need children beyond their own in whom to take an interest. It is simply a romantic notion that the love of a man and a woman is sufficient in itself to sustain their union. This same myth is applied also to the family, as though in their togetherness father, mother, and children can meet all their needs for intimacy within the family. God created the family not as a self-sufficient unit but as an organic part of the larger community. Families need each other even as persons need each other. We tend in our society to place too many demands upon the family to meet the needs of its members. This responsibility was meant to be shared by the community as a whole. The family simply cannot do it all alone.

In our nostalgia we look back on our rural past as the time of the extended family. That older rural society tended to be more stable than our present urbanized society. Yet not all rural cultures had extended families that functioned as such. It takes more than a common geography, work, history, and relatives to create an extended family; it also takes a spirit of love, affection, and caring.

The nuclear family, however, that is typical of our urbanized society is a step backward. By its very nature, the nuclear family undercuts the community it so desperately needs. In our illusionary need for privacy in our heavily populated societies, we have become our own worst enemies. We are, as Philip Slater's title suggests, actually pursuing loneliness (*The Pursuit of Loneliness*, rev. ed.; Beacon Press, 1976).

If the family needs community and community needs the family, where are they to find each other? We do not look to any romanticized period of our past to find the answer. We need only look to the nearest gathering place of the people of God. Your local congregation is now and has ever been the most likely place for your family to find community. This community of faith is a major resource in coping with mid-life crises.

OVERVIEW AND PERSPECTIVE

In this chapter, I have given an overview of how I see the mid-life crisis in Christian families. The chapters that follow will take up the specific factors referred to in this chapter and develop each in its application both to the generation and resolution of these conflicts.

Perhaps I have assumed that people in mid-life are bound to have a crisis. Many, of course, do. But this does not mean that you are abnormal if in mid-life you discover yourself without one. I seriously doubt, however, that a person can go through mid-life in our culture without having moments of sober reflection. This reflection, in turn, brings to the surface misgivings over aging and death, and raises anew the age-old questions about the meaning and purpose of life. Is your life and your marriage and your family what you want them to be? Or are you postponing their qualitative improvement to a vague tomorrow? How you respond to these reflections is bound to express itself in your family living. If you are interested in growing, in improving the quality of your family life regardless of how good it already is, in making the experience of mid-life the entrance into a more satisfying way of life, this book is for you, whether or not you are at this moment consciously in crisis.

2.Cultural Conditioning for Crisis

Our families are heavily influenced by the culture in which we live. This cultural influence isolates our families from the larger community. The Christian family is not immune to this isolation, for though it is not "of the world," it is still susceptible to the world's influence. What do we mean by "the world"? Obviously there are several meanings. In this context, however, I would define the world as the value system that sustains our culture—the values that give shape to what we mean by "making it" in our society, that define what we understand by winners and losers, by success and failure.

NOT OF THE WORLD BUT INFLUENCED BY IT

The conflict we have with the world is the counterpoint to the conflict we have within ourselves, a conflict described in the New Testament as that between the *flesh* and the *Spirit.* These are Biblical words for our sinful nature (flesh) in its conflict with the Spirit of God within us. In a similar way we are in conflict with our world: we are both of it and not of it. Yet it is not only that the world influences *us;* we also support and reinforce the world. As parents, we may at times even reinforce as well as mitigate the world's influence in our children. We bring the world into our homes. In mid-life the sharp difference between "*in* the world" and "not *of* the world"—between cultural values and those of the gospel of Christ—may become clearer. As we review our years of investment in the values of the world, we may realize that we have been "taken." This in itself constitutes a crisis.

What, then, are these values that support our culture? Philip Slater says you can tell what a culture really values by the choices people make when they have to choose. So long as we are not forced to get on one side or the other, many of us like to sit on the fence. Our values are revealed when we have to choose. Slater says that people of our culture prefer the values associated with competition over those associated with cooperation. This hardly needs documenting. We are a highly competitive people. Some competition stimulates us to do better. My wife and I signed up for a ten-day hike through the Welsh highlands. We thought we were in good physical condition, but the demands on us were more than we had anticipated. Had we been by ourselves, we would have quit early the first day. But not wishing to become lost in the Welsh woods we did not have that choice. By the end of the ten-day period we had discovered resources we did not know we had—and were keeping up with the others. The competition had been good for us. But there was also cooperation on that hike. The group stopped for us at intervals to catch up. Two young men waited for us at the gates and fences—all two hundred and fifty of them. In exchange we took their turn at dishes.

This is not an accurate description of much of the competition in our society. Not without reason do we refer to it as "cutthroat." People will cheat and even kill to "reach the top." Most of us stay within the law in our competitive strivings but violate the spirit of cooperation that sustains community. The toll that the pressures of competition take on our state of mind can be devastating. Instead of possessing the peace that passes understanding which Christ offers to us, we may know only the drivenness to excel. To excel means to excel over someone else. Each competitor, thus, becomes a threat to the self-esteem of the other. No wonder we hesitate to give advantages to others by cooperating with them.

These competitively oriented values easily infiltrate the life of the family. Lyndon Johnson's father used to rouse him out of bed in the morning by saying, "Get up, Lyndon, or every boy in the neighborhood will have a head start on you." Every other child is a competitior! When families get together and talk about their children, they often manifest the competition that exists even between families. The conversation can be quite one-sided as parents tell of the achievements, friendships, and honors associated with their children. Obviously the reporting is highly selective. Only rarely do people share the hurts, disappointments, failures that most children and their parents experience. Families are thus driven even more into isolation by the competitive pressures of our culture, and such isolation is the *last* thing our families need. Desperately trying to handle their problems by themselves because of the pride that competition engenders, these families may have to experience a crisis before they will expose their vulnerability by seeking help.

Another choice we tend to make, says Slater, is to value things—our material possessions, our property—over persons. The competitive spirit is also involved in this choice. Our possessions are symbols of our "making it" on the comparative scales of status and importance. Ironically this choice has a religious history. The early Puritans in seeking a sign of God's favor—and hence of their own salvation—saw in their material prosperity such a sign. How then to account for the many poor people who do not accumulate many possessions? Their poverty must be a sign of God's judgment! They are poor because they are lazy, shiftless, and perhaps even immoral. This kind of thinking is still with us. In a church bulletin dated April 1979, the question was raised concerning why there is poverty, disease, squalor, and drug addiction in our city slums. The answer given was that these slum dwellers are "slaves to sin and evil habits because they refuse the One who died to save and deliver them." The fact that these same "sins and evil habits" are not confined to the poor is ignored. The social stigma of poverty is reinforced with a moral stigma. In contrast to this negative judgment upon the poor is the Beatitude, "Blessed are you poor, for yours is the kingdom of God" (Luke 6:20).

Jesus had more to say on the subject. "A man's life does not consist in the abundance of his possessions" (Luke 12:15). In our culture, one's status, worth, rank, and rating may well depend on the abundance of things one possesses. It is often said that were Jesus to come to us today, he would be rejected by many churches. One reason for this rejection might be that he would be poor. "Foxes have holes, and birds of the air have nests; but the Son of man has nowhere to lay his head" (Luke 9:58). The hostility of the affluent toward the poor is revealed in their harsh judgments against people who are on welfare. They reflect the self-righteousness of the seventeenth-century Puritans when they say, "Let them work for their money as we do."

The values of a competitive society also move us to choose accomplishment over affection and personal intimacy. The result is that many families suffer from the effects of emotional isolation. The emphasis is on what we accomplish and not on who we are. Ironically, our sexual nature, through which our need for intimacy is expressed, is itself distorted into an accomplishment! We talk today about sexual *performance.* How we perform sexually supposedly reflects our worth as a person. Once we think of sexuality as a performance, it can actually be a barrier to intimacy, as it becomes susceptible to all the anxieties that go with our competitive value system. It may, therefore, be no coincidence that in mid-life, when we may be facing more realistically the limitations of aging, we may also be anxious over our sexuality: men anxious about their performance, women about their attractiveness. Since anxiety is counterproductive to what we are doing, it may actually create performance problems and even diminish our sexual attractiveness.

PRESSURES TO QUALIFY

Even as competition can be a good thing, so also can material possessions and achievement. The problem does not center in possessions or accomplishments, but in our attitudes toward them. It is a matter of our priorities. When we choose success over human values, we are undermining not only the security of our family relationships but also our own personal fulfillment. There are many "successful" persons today who are emotionally starved and whose families are malnourished in their need for intimate affection.

The value system of the world brings pressure upon us to qualify by its standards, and this pressure may crest in mid-life. According to our culture, personal worth must be proved. It is not something we are given; rather, it is something we must earn. So the pressure is on us to work at establishing our worth. Most of us get little assurance that we are "making it." Behind our determined efforts, consequently, is an underlying self-doubt which gnaws away at our self-esteem.

In mid-life the handwriting may be on the wall warning us that we are not likely to make it. Since we can no longer depend on an infinite future in which to hope, we look instead at the present. The sight may not be comforting. Oscar Brand's song may express our feelings.

> Can I go without a reason?
> How do I go from wherever I am?

As one fifty-year-old person put it, "I don't know whether I was ever any good, but I am worse now."

Suppose that you should be one of the "lucky" persons who in mid-life is considered to have "made it." This very awareness can bring additional pressures as well as additional doubts. You can *lose* it. Success today may be failure tomorrow. Also, you discover that rewards offered to those who "qualify" are not really that satisfying. In fact, when we realize what we may have sacrificed to achieve these rewards, their beauty may turn to ashes. Not only is the satisfaction quite transient, but also needs more germane to our humanity are left unsatisfied.

The world's values are essentially a cheat—they cannot give what they promise. If we give them highest priority, we have cheated ourselves. These values are off center from what is really meaningful in life. When we realize this, we may indeed face a crisis as the shallowness of our goals becomes increasingly manifest. We may feel like a busy executive who said, "If I could get away from all these demands that drive me bananas, I'd be better off." Yet it is not just the pressure of these demands that produces a crisis; it is also the judgment we experience for investing so much time and energy in them. In contrast to the Christ, our cultural values do not "have the words of eternal life" (John 6:68).

Culture in itself is not evil. In fact, culture is indispensable to community living. As people live together they develop mores, symbols, and traditions that constitute their culture, which in turn stabilizes their values. Within our overall culture there are subcultures and even countercultures, and all are in some form of interrelationship and in the process of change. As necessary as culture is to human society, however, all cultures, like the societies to which they are related, are human creations. Therefore, they contain the influence of the "world" even as their human contributors contain the influence of the "flesh." The community of faith must distinguish between the values of the culture in which it lives and those of the Kingdom of God, before which all cultures fall short. The danger is that the community of faith will become so acculturated that it will fail to discern the distinctions.

DISTRACTIONS AND EVASIONS

Pressures come upon us as we attempt to establish our personal worth on the basis of our cultural values. We are tempted toward various forms of addiction in order to relieve the stress. When I first taught pastoral care to theological students some twenty-five years ago, we focused primarily on female menopause when discussing mid-life crises. Today we focus instead on problems of the male. "What has happened to female menopause?" I asked in a conference with churchwomen. "Hormones and Valium," a woman answered, with tongue in cheek.

Yet the reference to Valium needs to be taken seriously. Prescription drugs are used increasingly to cope with the stresses of our time. Valium is perhaps the most popular. In a recent year, seven billion of these pills were taken. This represents a lot of hurt and turmoil. Valium, of course, can be a helpful drug in some instances. It can also become addictive. If such drugs are used as an escape from dealing directly with our tensions, we are postponing rather than evading a crisis.

By far the most common chemical distraction from our cultural pressures is alcohol. Alcoholism is our third most prevalent disease, heart disease and cancer coming before it. It cuts across all economic, social, and religious divisions. Alcohol is easily obtainable; it is available at most social gatherings. As one experiences its potential to change one's mood, to make one feel good, one is tempted to return to it for relief when pressures mount. Television dramas frequently model this way of escape, having their characters reach for a drink whenever they are frustrated or tense.

Television itself is for many people a nonchemical addiction. The average person watches six hours of television a day. The only activity most of us do more of is sleeping. Since this "addiction" affects children as much as adults, it is of particular concern to families. In my own community a local television station selected forty-five names at random from the telephone directory and offered those persons or families $500 if they would give up television for a month. Only twenty-seven accepted the offer. Of these, five were selected to be monitored.

These five families actually experienced withdrawal symptoms similar to those of chemical dependency. The television repairman who removed the sets said that the effect was like a death in the family. Although the experience was painful, some of these families discovered that while the children as well as the parents quarreled more without television, they were more likely to resolve their quarrels than before when something on television would distract them. Others said that out of boredom they learned to take initiative for entertaining themselves as families, and discovered their own creative potential.

Television offers us an illusionary world with which to identify when our own world is monotonous or painful. As we become addicted to this diversion, the people of the entertainment world become more "real" to us than the people we actually know. One of the children of a monitored family was asked what she would give up if she had to make a choice—television or talking with her father. She said, "Talking with my father."

The counterpoint to our need for entertainment is the way we magnify the people of the entertainment world.

They are the VIP's of our culture, enjoying disproportionate coverage in magazines and newspapers. On television talk shows, they are the most frequently interviewed. Their salaries are indicative of our adulation. The salary of one talk-show host is estimated at five million dollars a year. Professional athletics also pays its stars astronomical sums. We must need them badly, since it obviously is the public who makes such salaries possible. In addition, professional athletics provides a ready projection for our own competitive needs, as the anger we generate in our own frustrations is displaced in the "combat field" of the television screen. It can also provide a surrogate excitement that may be lacking in our lives.

Although television is for some an escape from the challenges of the real world, it can be and often is a good influence, providing an excellent medium for education, for entertainment, and for acquainting us with our world and its problems. It was, after all, a television station that conducted the experiment on television addiction. Public television in particular can contribute much to the enrichment of our lives.

For some of us, work is a respectable addiction. This is particularly true if our work is creative and open-ended. Work addiction has many rewards. These began early in our history, as the Puritans established the work ethic. Following the Calvinist doctrine of double predestination, they naturally desired signs that might indicate to which destiny they were predestined. Since they had to work hard to establish themselves in the new world, the success of this endeavor became for them such a sign.

When we are addicted to work, we not only avoid other

responsibilities and tensions but we also exploit what is otherwise a necessary and creative activity. Formed in the Creator's image we are by nature creative. Our work, whether inside or outside the home, provides an opportunity of expressing this creativity, as well as of contributing to the welfare of others in our life together. Not all jobs, however, permit one to be creative. Some jobs are primarily ways of making a living. These are not the jobs to which we become addicted. In these instances we have to find ways outside our work to express our creativity.

When our work is open-ended with creative opportunities, we can put so much of our time, energy, and concern into it that we have little of these left for other responsibilities. Our work then is a convenient distraction providing an escape from problems that require our attention, particularly in our families. Had we time and energy left to deal with these responsibilities, we would be without excuse if we neglected them. Our busyness is our protection, and therefore is potentially addictive.

Our work is also a way of qualifying in our society. While the Puritans used success in work as a sign of God's favor, in a more secular age we see it as a sign of societal favor. A responsible father is a good provider for his family. A responsible mother is a good homemaker who sacrifices so that her family can be comfortable. Of course, a subtle recompense is anticipated. The children, in turn, are to *do well* and thus be a credit to their parents. The persons whom we select as the father or the mother of the year are dependent partially for that honor on what their children have *accomplished.*

Work addiction in our culture is easy to justify. In harmony with our need to achieve status we justify our work by saying we need the money—so that our family can have the things that families are supposed to have. Work addiction, like other addictions, is hard on our health. The man—particularly the white man—in our culture seems to suffer most. He dies five years sooner on the average than women, often from diseases associated with stress. High blood pressure and coronary vascular disease are the two most common causes of death in middle-aged men, as personal crises are displaced into the body. It is not easy to qualify by the success of our work. Competition is heavy. We may feel forced into work addiction in order to keep our "head above water." Also, the means for competing may compromise our integrity. Repercussions from these external stresses are absorbed by our bodies when we do not take the time to deal with them directly.

MID-LIFE QUESTIONING

In mid-life we may question what heretofore we may have assumed. I have talked with middle-aged fathers who keenly regret not having given more of their time, energy, and creative concern to their families. I have talked with children who felt that their mothers were more concerned with being immaculate housekeepers than with relating intimately to their children. In mid-life we parents may realize that our involvement with our children is changing and that time may be running out. Even though this insight is sobering, it could be the beginning of our liberation from all of our protective addictions. Have we been on a treadmill seeking an unattainable goal? What is it we really want out of life? Or, to put it more humbly, to what is God calling us?

The rewards from our distractions and addictions, even from our work, may seem less fulfilling than we had assumed. In staying on top of things, we may have expressed a false sense of mastery over our destiny. In the pursuit of cultural goals by which we are deemed "successful" we lose sight of how fragile and temporary we really are. We need to hear the admonishment of James: "Come now, you who say, 'Today or tomorrow we will go into such and such a town and spend a year there and trade and get gain'; whereas you do not know about tomorrow. What is your life? For you are a mist that appears for a little time and then vanishes" (James 4:13–14).

Those who seek to control their futures find it hard to trust one another or even God. Relying primarily on our own efforts we are plagued by an underlying fear that we can't pull it off. It is time then to "consider the lilies of the field, how they grow; they neither toil nor spin; yet . . . Solomon in all his glory was not arrayed like one of these" (Matt. 6:28–29). In mid-life we become increasingly aware of our limits and subsequently aware of the folly of trusting primarily in our own controls. We are then in a position to recognize the only basis for security in a world over which we have so little control. Only as we trust in the Power beyond our own—our heavenly Father, who clothes the lilies—can we surrender this anxiety over tomorrow and "let the day's own trouble be sufficient for the day" (Matt. 6:34). Watergate conspirator John Dean said that he had become so absorbed in furthering his political career that he failed to "take time

to smell the flowers"—the *lilies* that could have taught him
other values.

When we see that mastery of our own destiny is an
illusion, we are then ready to confront our vulnerability.
This can be scary! Small wonder then that we are attracted
to another illusion—the cult of Superman. Someone surely
is invulnerable! Unfortunately or fortunately there are no
supermen; there are just other people like us. If we can let
go of our illusions, we may see our whole security system
caving in. Let it go! The old must die before the new can
come forth. Jesus speaks directly to our fear: "Do not be
anxious, saying, 'What shall we eat?' or 'What shall we
drink?' or 'What shall we wear?' Your heavenly Father
knows that you need them all" (Matt. 6:31–32). When the
old security system breaks down we are obviously in a crisis.
Christian faith provides a positive context within which to
view this crisis. The breakdown of the old can lead to the
breakthrough of the new! As we surrender our need to be
in control, we take the first step in learning to trust.

We are now ready to break out of the entrapment in
which our cultural values have placed us. Vic, for example,
started out so well as a young man that he never anticipated
that he would "level off." "At one time I was the youngest
regional director of our company," he said wistfully. "I was
obviously going places. Now in mid-life I'm not going any-
where! The promotion I wanted went to a darn kid. I've got
too much of my life invested in the company to leave. I'm
just trapped!"

Vic may be trapped as far as his promotional opportunities with the company are concerned, but he is not trapped

so far as his attitude is concerned. In fact, his frustration in climbing the ladder of occupational success provides him with an opportunity in mid-life to get a new—and better—set of values.

Vic's lament is not too different from that of Helen whose teenage daughter was using drugs. "How could this happen?" she asked. "Where did I fail as a mother?" Like Vic, she is hurt by the events that seem to put her down; like him, she has experienced a blow to her self-esteem. Yet a wounded pride, despite its pain, may be the way by which we discover humility. When our control systems break down we are confronted with our limits as human beings, not only in regard to our abilities but also in regard to our responsibilities. As J. B. Phillips has pointed out, when we assume too much responsibility for our own life as well as that of others, our God becomes too small. In the crises created by the collapse of our anticipations and assumptions, the way is prepared for God to reveal himself in all his fullness.

The end to our resources can prepare us for the resources that are beyond our own. With the collapse of our own powers also comes the collapse of the value system associated with these powers. Looking to the Power beyond our own means also looking to other values with which to give meaning to our lives. When our trust is in God, the assumption that our worth is established by how we do in our responsibilities at work or at home is seen to be false. The source of our worth is not in something we achieve but in something we have been given. Our worth is a gift of God. This realization places our achievements and our failures into a different perspective. We are liberated from burdens too heavy to bear. The conditions that lead to mid-life crises stemming from our adherence to cultural priorities lead also by that same token to the occasion—at times traumatic—for our emancipation from these priorities, together with their distorting effects on our lives.

3. Marriage and Family at Mid-Life

Our subject, mid-life crises in the Christian family, requires a look at the family—at your family. How are things going in your marriage? In what direction does your marriage seem to be moving? What kind of marriage do you—and your spouse—desire for the second half of your life? These questions are relevant to our concern, since mid-life crises often spill over into our family relationships. Three of the major crisis times for marriage occur in mid-life. The first is when the youngest child goes to school. This brings about a change in the life of the mother-wife. The critical issue is not simply that there is now extra time and energy, but the challenge to direct this time and energy into purposeful living. My wife went back to school when our youngest child began school. Others take a job outside the home. Some try other ways of rearranging their priorities. Whatever the course of action—or inaction—the wife-mother takes will have its effect on the marriage. Some husbands adjust well to these changes in their wife's activity; others have difficulty.

The next major crisis time for marriage is when adolescents rebel against parental authority. The change from a pleasant, adaptable child to a moody, defiant teenager can shake the family structure to its foundations. It can bring to the surface conflicts in the marital relationship that had remained latent until this time. Frustrated by their inability to cope, the spouses may blame each other for what is happening. "You're too hard on him," Mary said to Bob after a blowup with their sixteen-year-old son. "You don't listen to what he has to say before you begin yelling at him." Already smarting from the fracas, Bob counterattacked: "If you didn't spoil that kid like you do, I wouldn't *have* to holler at him!"

The third major crisis time is when the children have grown and left home. This provides the opportunity for the parents to take stock of their marriage. Has it a sufficient life of its own apart from the children? What will life be like with just husband and wife at home? For some, this is a time of depression and lostness. We parents can so identify with our children that their needs become our major concern. The emptiness of the "empty nest" may then reveal our own personal emptiness.

My wife and I have just completed our first year alone after thirty years of child-rearing. We both agree that it has been a good year. At times I was impressed with how quiet it was and really longed for some noise. But there are also opportunities for husband and wife to do things together and individually that they were not previously free to do. We have enjoyed these also.

Each of these three potential crisis periods is also a time

of opportunity—for positive as well as negative develop-
ments in a marital relationship. Even adolescent rebellion
can provide the occasion for husband and wife to seek help
for their family, and, in so doing, discover new ways for
cooperation in their common goals.

So let's take your marital pulse! How would you evaluate
the companionship dimension of your marriage? How often
do you share your feelings with your mate? Can you talk
about what is really important to you—your needs, desires,
hopes? Are you affectionate with each other? By affection
I mean not only how often or how satisfying your sexual
intercourse is but also how often you hug or tenderly touch
each other. Are there things you can't talk about without
getting into a quarrel? By this time you have probably accumulated your share of "old tapes." You can tell when you
are playing an old tape by the way you feel when you are
doing it, and by the fact that you are saying the very things
you really don't want to say.

Eric Berne has helped us to recognize what is going on
at such times by his earthy descriptions of these familiar
experiences. How better to describe our penchant for redo-
ing old quarrels than as "playing an old tape." Immediately
we can visualize our head full of old cassettes ready to play
when the button is pushed. Earlier, Sigmund Freud had
noticed this same tendency, calling it the *repetition compul-
sion. Old tapes* rings a clearer bell! Berne's other terms for
our unfortunate repetitions are equally pungent. We are
following a *script* written into our mind by our early experiences. The fact that we repeat rather than resolve our problems is an indication that we are *playing games.* But Freud

was right when he called such behavior *compulsive*. We feel trapped when we repeat behavior that our rational mind says is counterproductive.

Your marriage by now has acquired a history, having its own *roots*. Much of your past continues to repeat in your present. This can be useful as you build on your past in shaping your present. Your past can enrich your present. It can also distort it by being an obstacle to change and to growth. Are there unresolved issues coming out of your marital past that may be blocking your marital development, inhibiting the marital satisfactions that can come with the maturing years?

How has your marriage endured the role changes that have taken place in our day? In the small community in which my wife and I lived during the early years of our marriage, there was a well-known story about the local plumber who reacted to his wife's desire to get a job by saying, "The day you get a job I close the shop and go fishing." This reaction was viewed as a humorous illustration of one man's determination to be the breadwinner, in itself an admirable quality. Few in that community, including his wife, would have seen in such intransigence the stifling of his wife's self-development.

Since that day an increasing number of wives have acquired jobs in the community, and it has changed their roles within their marriage. The desire of any woman to have a life of her own apart from her family may be more pronounced in mid-life when family responsibilities decline. How did you perceive these roles when you entered into marriage? How do you perceive them now? Is there harmony between you and your spouse in this area?

During my first pastorate I encountered a young man who did not want his wife to come to gatherings at church if this meant that she could not be with him. "We love each other so much," he said, "that we do not want to be apart." Actually he left her alone many times for his work, but her primary duty was to be *there* when he was home. Her major purpose, in his mind, was to be his companion and comforter. Oddly enough, she did not seem to mind this lopsided arrangement. Today, she would probably be less accepting of such a role.

We all have problems over these role changes. I overheard a mother in her mid-thirties giving counsel to a young woman pregnant with her first child. Regretting that she had not stayed home with her small children, she said that if she had to do it over, she would do nothing else but mother them until they were in school. "But the times were against this," she said, "and I couldn't seem to affirm myself in the face of my job opportunity and the pressure from my boss."

Husbands have always had this problem. Not many would anticipate quitting work to be a father to their children—although some have worked part time in order to fulfill this responsibility. Rather, the expectation is that they take some time apart from their work to be with their children. At the same time, society expects fathers to be "good providers" and to be successful in their jobs. How, then, does one do both? Most often fathers solve this dilemma by going with the spirit of the times. Although there are pressures to serve both family and job, our society in effect says to the father,

Your job comes first! As one nineteen-year-old put it, "Mom reared us. Dad came home primarily to repack his suitcase." This choice, however, may be at considerable cost to the values that the father may come to cherish in mid-life. The sacrifice of family intimacy for job and career has been one of the hazards of being a male in our society. Obviously it is now also one of the hazards of being a liberated female.

Ironically, the changes in values and interests within the family may conflict with each other in mid-life. The husband and father who has worked hard in his early years to establish himself in his job may regret his lack of intimacy with his family in mid-life and may make direct overtures to his teenage children for their companionship. To his dismay they may not respond with much enthusiasm, for now they really prefer to be with their peers. In fact, they may not even want to be seen with their parents in public. Yet as small children they couldn't get enough of their father when his time and interest were severely rationed.

Rebuffed by his teenagers, the frustrated father reaches out as a husband to his wife. Surely she will respond, since it was she who previously complained that he was short-changing her in this regard. But in mid-life she may have become engrossed in a career outside the home and have neither the time nor the energy for the intimacy he now desires.

Because of changes like these Gail Sheehy says that the couple contract needs to be renegotiated in mid-life. Sore spots in the relationship that have been neglected because of the tensions inherent in them need now to be resolved. Otherwise the couple will project them into any new situation that resembles the previous traumas, and instead of moving into a fresh future, they will perpetuate a cyclic past. George, in the first chapter, believed he could not talk with his wife about their personal differences. She was recognized as a good mother and really also mothered him. Because she believed she knew what was best for her children and for her husband, she did not take his complaints seriously.

George may have encouraged his wife's maternal preoccupation in their earlier years because he felt more free then to devote himself to his work. Will Rogers, in his newspaper column for Mother's Day, 1930, wrote that the mother he knew the most about was his wife, since his own mother died when he was only ten years of age. Of his wife he said: "She has been for twenty-two years trying to raise to maturity four children; three by birth and one by marriage. While she hasn't done a good job, the poor soul has done all that a mortal human could do with the material she has had to work with." In mid-life a man may want something more than mothering from his wife, even if before this he was too busy for it. He now wants a wife, a companion, a soul mate.

George's wife, to the contrary, believed that since he had left the child-rearing to her and expected her to be the homemaker, he was now out of line in complaining that she was not fulfilling other roles such as that of a stimulating companion. Her world had not been as "stimulating" as his. While his days were filled with involvements with all sorts of persons concerned about all sorts of issues, she was confined to the world of her children, her neighbors, and her church. Each had developed differently in the course of their marriage and now the gap was apparent. Mid-life could have been the time to renegotiate their contract. Instead, it became the time for the dissolution of their marriage.

How Is It with the Children?

Let's take inventory concerning your children. How are they doing? Into what are they developing? Many of our homes have been "hit" by the drug problem. The availability of drugs to our children far exceeds that of a previous generation. They are also under strong peer pressures to be "sexually active." This comes not only from their peer group but also from the media. The media consistently convey the impression, explicitly or implicitly, that red-blooded, healthy young people *act out* their sexual desires. Moral, ethical, or religious directives for sexual activity are ignored. Those who resist acting out on their desires are portrayed as neurotically inhibited or sexually repressed. There is little societal support for young people to wait with their sexual activity until they can combine it with commitment.

We are becoming surfeited with our prolonged indulgence in sexual permissiveness. I was surprised recently to read the following statement in a university newspaper: "Sexual freedom has not delivered us to a utopia of fulfillment and security. By allowing intercourse without commitment to flourish, sexual freedom reveals its hidden paradox; the more we gorge ourselves without commitment, the emptier we feel. . . . You just can't lose by waiting. Haste, not chaste, makes waste." Whether or not we are "turning a corner" in our cultural permissiveness, the fact remains that young people today who are concerned about moral principles in regard to their sexual conduct may find themselves in a lonely position.

Those who have reared children recently know that it has been a difficult time also for parents. My mother more than once expressed to my wife and me how relieved she was that she was not rearing her children in our times. To experience rebellion from teenagers is nothing new for parents, but to experience it without the support of cultural values is a new experience. And it has been painful. As one father put it, "My daughter is confused about everything except that her parents don't know anything!" Authorities in the field have much to say about dealing with adolescent rebellion, but it may be frustrating as well as helpful. "We need to take a balanced attitude as our children battle restraints," says one such authority. "If we offer no restraints, they will do battle with the restraints of the schools and community. That can mean trouble. And if we are overly restraining at home, we encounter dangers such as early marriages in order to escape, or other acts of desperation, such as running away, drunkenness, or reckless driving." Needless to say, this "balanced attitude" which the psychiatrist recommends is not only difficult to achieve but at times difficult even to ascertain.

Adolescent rebellion seems to strike capriciously in families—and among families. One child may rebel with self-destructive vehemence, while other children in the same family experience only a mild or even positive form of rebellion. Family counselors point out that each child in a family has a different position in the family and with the parents. While each particular system of relationships contributes its own influence in a person's behavior, it cannot by itself explain why this person behaves as he or she does. Others in similar positions in similar environments may respond differently. Why? Why also do some families have the problem of excessive rebellion while others do not? Is the afflicted family an inferior family? This is what the parents fear. But any objective evaluation of famlies would find such a general judgment hard to substantiate.

Adolescent rebellion in regard to alcohol and other drugs, sexual behavior, school or church involvement, and violent altercations over parental rules is only one form of family frustration. Not all children worry their parents by their late hours or their "bad" company. Some children withdraw from their peers or are otherwise left out of their own social milieu. Some also withdraw even from their families. "Mary spends too much time in her room—and I don't know what to do about it. She doesn't seem to have any close friends. I'm worried about her." This lament by Mary's mother is not over the usual adolescent stereotype. Mary's withdrawal to her room indicates her loneliness. Yet she resists overtures of her family to help her. "We don't have any shouting matches like I have had with my other children," her mother continued. "I actually think I can handle the fighting better."

Mary's mother is like most parents in our activitist culture. We have a difficult time understanding and accepting youngsters who retreat into themselves. Yet it is the way in which some adolescents attempt to cope with their confused feelings and hurts.

LIMITATIONS OF PARENTAL ROLE

Because of the problems that they may be experiencing with their children, parents at mid-life tend to become increasingly aware of their limitations as parents. Whatever myth they may have entertained about parental powers is short-lived. In our untested innocence we may have been quite critical toward older parents. "I would never put up with such shenanigans from their kid as they do!" One of these older parents shared with me his reaction to a similar criticism by a young neighbor woman over the noisy behavior of his adolescent son and his friends. "Wait till her kids get a little older," he said. "She'll see how different it is than when her child was a three-year-old."

The young woman's response is typical of the way we react to disruptive teenagers. We are angered and convinced that they need a forceful demonstration of parental control. When the shoe is on the other foot, we may not be so sure of our mastery. Force—especially physical force—has its limits. Other forms of force may also be ineffective. "For that smart remark, you'll not get the car for a month," roared Dave's father. "Keep your old car," Dave shot back. "I wouldn't use it if you gave it to me!" Where do we go from here? What happens when our "club" is resisted? Defied? It can be a frustrating moment in any parent's life. If our pride is invested in this power struggle, it is also a humiliating moment. When confronted by the police regarding her child's behavior, a shaken mother replied, "I'm sorry, but I have to admit that I can no longer control her."

To recognize our powerlessness can be a sobering awareness. When force no longer works, we are introduced once again to our creatureliness. We need help! Otherwise we will continue on a collision course with our children. The collapse of our controls, however, need not be disastrous. Although it marks the end of one way of doing things, it may also mark the beginning of new—and perhaps better—ways. Mid-life may be the time to renegotiate the parent-child contracts also, as a preparation for the relationship soon to come when the children will be young adults.

Most family irritations have their humorous side. Consider how television uses these family tensions for situation comedy. How many of us have laughed at Archie Bunker's livid countenance during the frequent quarrels of the Bunker family? When we experience our own family quarrels, however, we rarely see the humor. Instead, we are overly serious and overly anxious. If we could relax enough to see the humor, we could be liberated from our usual script and effectively change the course of the dialogue.

Henri Nouwen says that children are more like guests than possessions. Parents, then, are hosts. We are not responsible for our guests, but we are responsible for hosting them while they are with us. Does this seem like an odd description of the parental role? Considering the guilt trip that society lays on parents for their children's behavior, I imagine that it may even seem ridiculous. What, we may ask, does a Catholic priest like Nouwen know about rearing children? It may, however, be a comforting analogy. We may be accepting too much responsibility for our children as well as too little. It may be a relief to have some of this responsibility reapportioned.

Assume for the moment that we *are* hosts to our children. While this may alter our usual image of parental responsibility, hosts do have a role: they respond to the needs of their guests. What does this mean in reference to our parental role? A clue may lie in the fact that we need ultimately to let our children go. As Nouwen puts it: "It indeed is hard to see our children leave after many years of much love and much work to bring them to maturity, but when we keep reminding ourselves that they are just guests who have their own destination, which we do not know or dictate, we might be more able to let them go in peace and with our blessing. A good host is able not only to receive his guests with honor and offer them all the care they need but also to let them go when their time to leave has come." (Henri Nouwen, *Reaching Out: The Three Movements of Spiritual Life*, p. 58; Doubleday & Co., 1975.)

The idea that children are guests of their parents contrasts with the idea that children belong to their parents. Love can easily slip into possessiveness. We have mental pictures of what our children should be like or how they should develop and these pictures may be a dominant factor in our relationship to them. Whatever gaps exist between these pictures and the real child may disappoint us. Spoken or unspoken, this disappointment is often picked up by our children and they feel inadequate—put down. It is probably this judgmental attitude that the Scripture writer is concerned about when he admonishes parents not to discourage their children (Col. 3:21).

As guests, our children would have more freedom to be who they are. There would also be more room for them to have God for a parent. It is easy for parents to assume that God has the same anticipations for their children as they do. Yet it is the mark of the creature to recognize his or her difference from the Creator, and to permit the mind of God to be something other and beyond the projections of the minds of his creatures. If we are to be relieved of assuming too much responsibility for our children, we need to surrender to God the possessiveness that can contaminate our love. Then we can learn to see our children as they are without having to compare them to some preferred image in our heads. It is amazing how much more we see in our children when we are not looking through the lenses of our preconceived preferences. As we surrender our possessiveness, we can learn to trust our children, and even more, to trust that God is involved with our children, although in ways that may be hidden to us. When we trust in the power beyond our own we can observe our children as they are and grow in our appreciation of them.

DEALING WITH OLD TAPES

Although it is good to see what needs to be done to improve our relationship with our children, old tapes in our head may continue to play, so that the desired changes seem remote. Some of these tapes may come from our own days as teenagers, except that the roles now are reversed: we take the role of our own parents in our relationship to our children. Perhaps you have noticed that you may say the same words to your child that your parent used to say to you, even though you didn't like those words then and your children don't like them now. The imprint is in our minds and we follow the same script, although we have changed parts. One good thing about these reenactments is that we understand our own parents better and have more compassion for them than we did when we were on the other end of the transaction.

Other more recently cut tapes may also be replayed especially with younger children. They not only get the outgrown clothing of their older siblings, but also receive the reverberations of their parents' relationship with them. The comparisons with which we approach our younger children are often based on our prior experience with our older children. By mid-life we have established certain patterns in dealing with our children. We either expect our younger children to follow these same patterns or we live in fear that they will. In either case the younger ones may sense the shadow from their older siblings in their relationship with their parents.

It is difficult to perceive reality as it is. We tend to project our past impressions upon it along with the anxieties that go with these. Some of these projections are necessary in order to interpret what we are receiving. Otherwise we would not profit from our experiences or achieve the wisdom that may come to us with the accumulation of years. When these projections are based on past conflicts that have remained unresolved, however, we may misinterpret more than interpret. So we need to be flexible about our interpretations, separating actual data from our overactive emotions and desires. The more we can dispense with our arbitrary way of evaluating what we see in our children by standards that are culturally conditioned, and instead see simply the children, the more we will experience spontaneous affection for them.

HELP THROUGH MEDITATION

Most of us need help in breaking the repetitive and counterproductive patterns of our family relationships. Instead of compulsively playing the old tapes when our emotions are aroused, we need to cut new ones that more realistically fit the moment. Although we are creatures of habit, we can also create new habits. Even as habits are formed by repetition, so they cease to be habits when they are not repeated. When we break the repetition by responding differently in a family situation, and repeat this response on the next occasion, we are on the way toward forming a new habit.

To form new habits in communication is easier to describe than to accomplish. As one frustrated spouse said, "When I'm irritated I have knee-jerk reactions rather than ideas for doing things differently." We may need the help of others, particularly other families. Marriage Encounter is available in most communities, as is Parent Effectiveness Training. I recommend both from personal experience. Your pastor, local social agency, or community counseling service can provide the needed information concerning these and other group-oriented opportunities. Sharing with other families helps us to realize that we are not alone in our problems. It also provides the support we need—and suggestions—as we work for improvement in our family living.

There is also something that you and your family can do on your own. Changes may begin within ourselves before they become manifest in our relationships. The practice of meditation is a way of beginning with oneself. Meditation has a long history in the Christian tradition, although it has received recent impetus in our midst from Eastern religions. Though our Western culture may have responded to Eastern versions of meditation as something new, the Gospel accounts of Jesus show that prayer and meditation were very much a part of his life. He not only practiced this discipline but went to considerable lengths to secure the right time and place. He would climb a mountain for the place or rise up "a great while before day" for the time. It was not unusual for him to pray all night. "In these days he went out to the mountain to pray; and all night he continued in prayer to God" (Luke 6:12).

Meditating is a particular kind of praying; it is praying with our total person. Instead of speaking words as we usually do in prayer to God, we *listen* to words and mentally *picture* our petitions. Meditation, thus, is the focusing of our imagination in the presence of God.

We begin meditation by consciously relaxing our body and slowing the pace of our mind. Personally, I prefer to sit in a straight, hard chair, with my feet on the floor and my arms resting on my thighs. When we are physically relaxed and mentally still, our spirit seems more receptive to the Spirit of God. Prayer begins by our listening to the Spirit. The Spirit speaks through the Word—the Scriptures. In your meditation I would suggest you choose a favorite Scripture verse that you have memorized and focus on it, letting the Spirit speak to you through it. As an example, take Prov. 3:5–6: "Trust in the Lord with all your heart, and do not rely on your own insight. In all your ways acknowledge him, and he will make straight your paths." As you listen to these words, picture yourself as trusting in God in regard to your marriage and family relationships—and not relying on your own insights (interpretations). See yourself acknowledging his presence in the most unlikely situations—such as in moments of irritation or disappointment with yourself, your spouse, or your children. Notice the difference it makes in your own behavior at these times. Then envision your paths straight: your confusion is dispersed and you are letting the Spirit direct your ways in your family concerns.

To reinforce this Biblical directive in your life, select a particular frustration tape that you tend to play in an irritated moment, despite your desire not to do so. Actually see yourself in such a moment, but then respond differently. You may even imagine yourself turning off the "tape recorder" and speaking the way you really want to speak. In this way you break fresh ground in your mind by letting the Spirit direct you. At the same time, your mental picture is a prayer to God that you actually will behave in this manner in these circumstances. Inwardly say *amen* ("So let it be").

Prayer is also intercession for others. Suppose you are concerned about one of your children. The child may be giving indications of problems at school or with peers or with his or her religious faith. In meditation you picture your child as overcoming these problems. See the child confident at school, at ease with peers, and inwardly secure in the love of God. Intercession for your spouse would be expressed in a similar manner. Include also your marital relationship. Picture your marriage as growing in intimacy, in trust, and in enjoyment. Picture you and your spouse enjoying companionship, sharing deeply each other's feelings and concerns. Feel your affection in that moment for your spouse and for each of your children. Picture yourself hugging them and them hugging you.

It may take a "leap of faith" to visualize in this manner what God can do in your life and in the life of your family. What you actually see in the daily occurrences in the family may not support such envisioning. So your meditative visualizing is an act of faith—of responding to God's promises. God not only invites us but directs us to ask for help in our needs. Meditation is a way of asking that also prepares us to receive.

Besides being a form of prayer, meditation is also a conditioning exercise. By repeating in our minds as a regular discipline the ways in which we experience God's call to change and to grow, we are preparing ourselves for these changes in our behavior. What we "see" ourselves doing in our meditation we may actually do as a result. We practice this same kind of discipline in our church services. Besides being a way of worshiping God, the repetition of formal or informal worship patterns is also a way by which we are conditioned to grow more into the likeness of God. Regular attendance at worship services, therefore, as well as a daily discipline of prayer and meditation, should be looked upon as our obligation not only to God but also to ourselves.

In our efforts to improve our family life, we should not delude ourselves with perfectionist fantasies. "Victories" are now and then rather than once and for all. As participants in a fallen humanity we shall continue to have conflict between the flesh and the Spirit, in which we are absolved of judgment by God's covenant of forgiveness. But there will be victories! They are made possible by the forgiveness we receive for our failures.

4. The Specter of Aging and Death

"What time is it?" As I asked this I received the answer that it was twelve after twelve in the afternoon of June 2, 1979. By the time you read this, a lot of minutes, hours, days, weeks, and months will have gone by. What is time? A fascinating enigma! We are tyrannized by time, amazed by it, victimized by it, and challenged by it. Time has to do with beginnings and endings. Time itself has a beginning and an ending: we speak of the "dawn of time" and the "end of time." In the meantime—the "intervening time" between the beginning and the ending—time runs its erratic course. Sometimes it *flies* and other times it *drags*. A desired event may seem far in the future. Children, anticipating Christmas, may jump up and down with excitement, saying, "I can't wait! I can't wait!" But they do wait, and the desired event arrives—and then it is past. Soon Christmas was a week ago, and then a month ago. Finally the time will come when "our time is up." There is an end.

This end to time in our own lives is connected with the aging process, a process marked by birthday celebrations.

But we don't just celebrate them, we count them. We also celebrate anniversaries—wedding anniversaries, for example. We not only count them, but even name some of them —paper, wooden, silver, golden. There are other anniversaries that we do not celebrate, but remember nevertheless. This day, June 2, 1979, is also the sixth anniversary of our oldest daughter's funeral. Tears come easy to this memory. Our birthdays also take on an ambiguity in mid-life. We know their number is limited, and when they begin to pile up, we become more aware that there is a last one somewhere up ahead. So in mid-life some of us don't like to mention our birthdays. As long as no one knows it is your birthday, you won't be asked which one it is.

In spite of our reluctance to acknowledge our aging, our society is highly age conscious. When Margaret Chase Smith was running for reelection as senator from Maine, she lamented that newspapers identified her not simply as Senator Margaret Chase Smith, but as Senator Margaret Chase Smith, 65. Rarely does the press relate any news about a person without stating that person's age, at least as young, middle-aged, or elderly. As a culture we are highly sensitive to the passage of time. "Hurry or you won't make it!" could be our slogan.

While we measure time objectively by our watches and calendars as the earth rotates around the sun, there is also a subjective measurement of time. Some minutes seem longer than others, some days shorter. "I thought this day would never end!" or "I don't know where the time has gone!" The weeks, months, and years seem to go faster as we get older. The years from mid-life on seem literally to gallop. The closer we come to running out of time, the faster it seems to go.

Human beings would like on occasion to "stop the clock." One of the more remembered stories of the Old Testament is that of Joshua praying for more time in the midst of a battle and "the sun stood still." Most of us would at least like to slow it down.

As a person in mid-life, you are now at an age that you would previously have considered old. It is amazing how differently we view these ages once we arrive at them. When you were "bright and bushy-tailed" at twenty-one, you probably couldn't imagine yourself being all of fifty or even forty years of age. How about now? Can you imagine yourself as seventy or eighty years old? Although we know we cannot do anything about this "ever-rolling stream" that bears us all away, we can still feel depressed or worried about it. This worry may persist in the back of our minds while we are involved in our daily pursuits even when we appear to others to be lighthearted and gay. We feel the pressure from the speed at which time seems to be moving, as well as anxiety over where it is taking us.

You may need a perspective that has come to terms with the end of time as you enter the second half of life. Though death is an indigenous part of life, even the elderly may not be ready for it. An elderly faculty colleague stricken with a terminal illness lamented that he had so many projects that he was not going to be able to finish. I was young then and not as prepared as I am now to understand such a lament. Unless one is terminally ill, death is usually unanticipated. The litany of the liturgical churches contains the petition, "From an unprepared and evil death, good Lord, deliver us."

Preachers warn us to "get our house in order," so that the hour of death does not find us unprepared.

The perspective on life that we need for its second half can come to us through our faith in God. Where previously we may have used our faith as a support for accomplishment and achievement, we now need it as a support for *quality* of life. When we refer to the second half we are reckoning with the *quantity* of life. Quality is determined by what happens within the quantity. While we can do nothing about the fact that all life ends in death, we can do something about the quality of life *before* it ends in death.

This realization gave birth to the movement Make Today Count. Orville Kelly, terminally ill with cancer and father of young children, decided that though he had little control over the quantity of life left to him, he could do something about the quality of that life. After a family conference in which his approaching death was frankly faced, the decision was reached to work together for quality in life. "I will have good days and bad days," said Kelly, "but let's make every day count regardless." The result was a marvelous change in the quality of life in his family. He described the experience in a Burlington, Iowa, newspaper and received many inquiries from terminally ill persons and their families. The result was the initiation of the organization Make Today Count.

While some persons are terminal with a disease for which medical science has no cure, the rest of us are terminal because our bodies are destined to age and die. Therefore we can apply Orville Kelly's insight into life's quality to our own lives, though we have no known terminal illness. I prefer to say, *"Let* today count," because I believe that God is in our midst giving us grace to enhance the quality of our lives. But he won't force his grace on us; we can resist it. In fact, we *do* resist it as we seek first the values of our production, achievement, and success-oriented culture instead of those of the Kingdom of God. Instead of resisting God's overtures, it is possible for us to respond to them in faith. It is a matter of *letting* happen what God's grace can *make* happen.

In a psalm that refers to the limited quantity of human life, there is a prayer for the quality of these years. "Teach us to order our days rightly, that we may enter the gate of wisdom" (Ps. 90:12, NEB). One might paraphrase this prayer by saying, "Teach us rightly to prioritize our days, for wisdom is essentially a right ordering of priorities." The accumulation of years does not in itself lead to wisdom. "There is no fool," we say, "like an old fool." But the years can lead to wisdom if we listen to them and learn from them. Although we learn much from education that can be applied as wisdom, wisdom is not the same as education. There is no fool also like an educated fool.

Wisdom is the knowledge of values that comes through one's own experience. In mid-life we are in a prime position to grow in wisdom. With the experience of the first half of life behind us, and the sharper perception of our limits in the life ahead, we know better than before what determines quality of life.

The Trauma of Aging

The marks of aging are not easy to ignore. As they appear, they can take their toll on our mental state. Each can produce its own trauma: graying hair, thinning hair, increase of weight, wrinkling of the skin on face and hands, the lines, jowls, bags, double chin, and other unwelcome additions to the face. The cosmetic industry supplies coverings for most of these. Formerly it was preponderantly women who used these, but the industry now is appealing to an increasing number of men. In an economic world that casts out the aged, it seemingly is to one's advantage not to *look* old. Advertisements for various commodities appeal to our desire to look younger and feel younger. We are obviously attempting to slow something down—perhaps even to deny it altogether. The trauma of aging is based on the foreboding that one will soon be "over the hill."

Our society apparently perceives no advantages in growing older. The end of the route is especially repugnant. Even worse than being "over the hill" is to enter a nursing home. Here we see the epitome of all the disadvantages in becoming old. If you have visited one of these homes, you probably said to yourself: "Not I. Spare me this. I'd rather die first." The residents may have said something similar a few decades earlier. How, then, do they end their days here? These homes, of course, differ widely in quality, depending largely on what one is able to pay, but none can exclude the grim atmosphere of segregation and dependency.

We tend to segregate the elderly. We do this with most of the human conditions that we do not want to see. By institutionalizing the retarded, the disabled and disfigured war veterans, the chronically ill, and the deteriorated elderly, and by segregating the poor, the racially different, and the culturally deprived, we can more easily forget that they exist. If these people were living in our own neighborhoods or gathering in our own churches, we would be reminded not only of their existence but also of our involvement in their plight and of our own possible destiny.

That destiny may become ominously clear in mid-life. Your parents are growing older and may be approaching the time when they can no longer live by themselves. What to do? You may help make the decision. If you have been through it, you know how difficult it is. If communities worked together to assist the elderly, many of them could remain in their own homes much longer. Some homes for the aged are extending their services into the community, so that older people may not need to enter the home. Yet the predominant impression seems still to be that the elderly who need help should go in to a home. We surely need nursing homes and homes for the elderly. We also need communities and congregations who accept responsibility for the elderly in their midst, and who work together to keep them interdependent members of the community as long as possible.

Not only does the aging process lead to death, but death may come slowly. The advanced stages in old age deterioration are the farthest cry from our society's image of beautiful people. Ernest Hemingway's portrayal of the macho man, abounding in physical virility and endurance, virtually invulnerable, is difficult to conceive in the context of old age. It was hard for America to see macho actor John Wayne stricken by disease and unable to whip the Big C. It was hard for Hemingway himself to experience the marks of aging. He had planned to end his life before he was ravaged by age and he did. As an old man, Edward G. Robinson, the actor known for his portrayal of the tough, indomitable Little

Caesar, spoke pathetically about the humiliation and indignities that come with old age.

Because of aging parents, people in mid-life often get caught with unanticipated responsibilities. Our parents in their increasing inability to cope for themselves may require more and more of our time and energy—and concern. We thought we had left our parents to cleave to our spouse, but now our parents need *us*. At the same time, children whom we had thought had left home to be on their own may need us also. A daughter may experience the trauma of divorce and be left with the custody of small children. For her to work, she may need her parents' assistance in caring for her children. Or a son back from a hitch in the armed services may have difficulty getting a job and want to live at home for a while. But it may not be the same. Some of his later acquired ways may not fit with the traditional mores of the home. The couple who are caught in the middle may begin to "feel their age." Mid-life is not the break from family responsibilities they had anticipated.

Our first brush with death is usually with a grandparent. Many persons who are middle-aged have already experienced the death of a parent, a sibling, a child, or a good friend. The older we become, the more likely we are to experience such losses. Besides the pain of grief, they remind us of our own impending death. Life includes death and we need to become reconciled to this reality.

For the life we have yet to live, we need support from others. Each human relationship is unique; therefore each loss irreplacable. Yet the place it filled need not remain empty. My mother at eighty-three had as many friends as she did at forty-three. She had the ability—or was it the motivation?—to develop new friendships to replace those which death had taken. Most of these were younger, some far younger, than she. Yet the friendships were no less intimate or meaningful than those which she had lost.

In spite of our foreboding over aging and death, we rarely deal with them directly in mid-life as problems. Instead, we deal with their symptoms. George, the husband who wanted out of his marriage, never spoke directly about his "bothers" over aging. Instead, he talked about seeking his fulfillment before it was too late. What is "too late"? These are terror words to persons obsessed by the fear of aging. George's desperation was shown in his remark, "No matter who gets hurt, I've got to do it!"

Tom showed his anxiety over aging in a different way. He was a workaholic. The more years he lived, the more compulsively he worked at his job. His work distracted him from worry. But more importantly, his addiction was a way of demonstrating how indispensable he was. It didn't make sense rationally (people are not especially rational when pursued by dread). If he faced his fears directly, he might come to a more rational way of dealing with them.

Jane's way of coping with aging anxiety was more obvious than Tom's. Although she was in her mid-forties, she continued to dress like a teenager. She was especially thrilled when people said that she and her nineteen-year-old daughter looked like sisters. Not only her dress and her hairdo but also her way of speaking and her behavior placed her in the same age bracket. Her daughter's initial amusement with her mother's attempt to stay young had turned to annoyance. She had enough competition among her peers without having her mother also in that role. One night her mother was flirting in a subtle way with some of the daughter's friends at a picnic. The daughter said, "Mother—for heaven's sake!—why don't you act your age!"

In spite of these aberrant ways of coping with aging, mid-life can be a time to invest in the process of *positive* aging. If we take off our cultural blinders, we will see that there are actually advantages to aging. A great deal of the negative perspective on aging is culturally conditioned. Older people are arbitrarily placed outside the mainstream of community life. They are prevented from making meaningful contributions to society or even to their own families. This loss of worth—loss of being needed—leads also to the loss of purpose. People need a reason to get up in the morning. If they lack this reason, they may soon forget what day it is. What does it matter?

Older people are informed in no uncertain terms by the business and medical worlds that the degenerating symptoms of aging are inevitable, irreversible, and universal. The implication is that one's value to society declines with these symptoms. So it is only right that older people should retire —not just from business, but from life. Even in mid-life when we forget something or feel achy and sore, we may say, "I must be getting old!" We are programmed in this direction by the assumptions of our day. It takes a lot of ego strength to refuse to follow the prescribed aging path.

Now is the time to invest in your old age. As people become older, they tend to become "more so," more fixed in the patterns they were following. Obviously it pays to take a good legacy of behavior patterns into old age. A friend of mine in his early eighties laments that had he known he was going to live so long, he would have taken better care of himself. At first this struck me as hilarious. How would he live into his eighties had he not taken good care of himself! But the fact is that he could! It *is* possible to abuse one's body or mind or spirit and still live to be old. It is just as possible to take good care of one's body, mind, and spirit and die young. There are no guarantees in a life full of contingencies. So, my friend is right after all. He probably would be better off in his elderly years if he had taken better care of himself in his early and middle years—physically, mentally, and spiritually.

COMING TO TERMS WITH DEATH

To invest positively in the aging process our first need is to come to terms with death, specifically our own death. Our life has a terminus. Its duration is not much different now from what it was in Old Testament times, when the psalmist wrote, "The years of our life are threescore and ten, or even by reason of strength fourscore" (Ps. 90:10). One may get the impression that we are living longer today because of the recent advances in medical science. Actually we are not. It is just that *more* of us are living longer. The average life-span of the first seven presidents of the United States was 79.2 years. It probably would have been more had not Washington, the one who died youngest, at sixty-seven, been severely weakened in his illness by the medical practice of bleeding. Through the advances of medical science, today in the developed nations a greater percentage of people reach advanced years. Yet the quality of life for these years has actually deteriorated. In mid-life we need to be concerned about the quality of life we will have if we reach old age.

How do you feel about your own death? Actually the question is not whether you will die, but when and how. So says our reason. Yet we find it hard to accept the fact that we will come to an end. There is a subrational, gut-level reaction that says, "It can't happen to me." The reason for this ambiguity is that death is both natural and unnatural. Life as we know it needs death. Not only human beings die; all forms of life die. We can't have births without deaths, beginnings without endings. Because births are getting ahead of deaths, we are having a population problem. Should this continue, starvation, environmental pollution, or wars of survival may increase the deaths until we reach an equilibrium.

As necessary as death is to life, the thought of our own death can seem most unnecessary. Even as we cannot remember our beginning, we have trouble anticipating our ending. Something in our own self-awareness seems to imply that we are immortal. While we would be too rational to acknowledge this in any questionnaire concerning our beliefs, our actions often indicate that we are laboring under this illusion.

Despite our ambiguity regarding our own death, two things are certain. The first is that at mid-life our youth and young adulthood are over, and for our culture these constitute the golden age. When something is gone that we value, we grieve over the loss. This is a natural wholesome process in resolving the loss. Mourning has a purpose: "Blessed are those who mourn, for they shall be comforted." Grieving is potentially healing. But in order to grieve in a healthy way one needs to express one's feelings to another, focusing directly on the sense of loss. This is particularly difficult for men in our culture. Two illustrations out of three that I gave regarding persons projecting their anxiety over aging into other symptoms were male. This was not coincidence. Because they have less pressure on them to be strong and tough, women can be more direct in expressing their feelings of loss. Direct dealing with our grief over the loss of our youth will help us grow in our ability to let it go. As we are comforted in our mourning over the past, our anxiety over the future—over aging and death—will also abate.

But the task is not simply a personal one—it is also cultural. Some cultures glorify mid-life; others, old age. This leads to other kinds of problems. Since our culture is fixed on youth, the values associated with growing older are deemphasized. We need to challenge the youth-success-production emphases of our culture. We may have survived being taken in by these values in the first half of life, but they will be destructive to us if they are followed in the second half. They simply do not lead to quality living, which is necessary for the second half. Even our games are based on competitive and acquisitive life-styles. I am not referring only to the commercialization of athletics but also to the parlor games we play with our children. Take Risk for example: each player wages war on the other in a battle for control of the world. The moral and ethical milieu is that of the third temptation of Jesus in which he is offered "all the kingdoms of the world and the glory of them" (Matt. 4:8). Or Monopoly. The gross national product mentality is dramatized on the game board as we progress from houses to hotels and from one property to conglomerates, as the prosperity of the winners leads to the financial ruin of the losers.

These games are lots of fun. We've played them innumerable times in our family. But they and others like them are based on a value system that has little relevance to that of our Christian faith. So for an occasional balance I suggest that you play the Ungame with your children. Devised by Rhea Zakich as a game for her family, the Ungame is aptly named. There are no winners or losers, no accumulation of points, territory, or houses, no difficult decisions concerning whether or not to send your opponent back to start, and not even a prescribed ending. The Ungame is played like other games: players throw dice and move their own "pieces" on a board. But these simply determine the card you select, which in turn provides a specific way of sharing yourself with the others. You may learn something about your family members from the Ungame that they might not otherwise share with you. Also one can always pass. The game will introduce your children—or grandchildren—to the fun of sharing and listening. Since they are inevitably receiving double signals from the adult world about values and priorities, it is good for them to have at least one family game that reinforces the values associated with those of the Christian faith.

The second certainty is that death is ahead for all of us. A life that is realistic and at the same time positive must therefore be a life that has come to some sort of harmony with death. Those of us in mid-life must choose values that take our mortality seriously, for as the Scripture puts it, "here we have no lasting city" (Heb. 13:14). These values that we select must also take seriously the symptoms and symbols of death, especially disease, tragedy, and failure. Those who suffer with these symptoms often cry out: "Where is God in all of this? How can he permit such tragedies to happen?" While this is an expression of healthy grieving, it does not yet deal with a distinctly Christian concept of God. Our God, whose own Son was most cruelly and unjustly killed, also suffers. Our faith centers in a Christ who was crucified—who in agony asked to be spared such a death—and was not. Yet our faith does not end with a crucified Christ. The symptoms and symbols of death as well as death itself are transcended by the resurrection. The cross is followed by the empty tomb. "We seek the city which is to come" (Heb. 13:14).

Because of its realistic approach to death (the crucified Christ) and its positive approach to life (the empty tomb), our Christian faith provides the potential both to affirm life and to accept death. Kenneth Vaux points out that, on the one hand, human beings tend to have a love for life coupled with an underlying fear of death, and, on the other, a subconscious fear of life and a yearning for death. This ambivalence is an obstacle both to our affirmation of life and to our acceptance of death. Yet it is Christian neither to abhor death nor to deem it natural. Human beings created in God's image do not accept death as a natural dénouement of their lives. Yet death as the enemy of life is overcome through Christ's death and resurrection. On the basis of our Christian beliefs we can make value choices that are both positive and realistic. "The authentic will to live," says Vaux, "contains a willingness to die" (Kenneth Vaux, *Will to Live, Will to Die*, p. 133; Augsburg Publishing House, 1978). We can bring death into harmony with life in our lives because its "sting" is removed through the death and resurrection of Christ and not because fear and pain are gone.

FUTURE ORIENTATION VS. HOPE FOR THE FUTURE

As Christians we have hope for this life and for its eternal fulfillment that transcends death. The hope in either case is related directly or indirectly to the resurrection of Christ and through this event to our own resurrection. While we associate the latter resurrection with our future, it also has a realization dimension in our present. Paul describes the Christian as one who has been "brought from death to life" (Rom. 6:13). John describes eternal life as a present possession, given to us through knowing "him who is true" (I John 5:20). Belief in the resurrection irrevocably unites the present with the future and the future with the present. Because we believe in the resurrection we have hope in the present, and because we experience resurrection in the present we have hope for the future. The Christian faith ties together the tenses so that each is interdependent with the others. Through the resources of our faith we can focus on the present even as we profit from the past and experience the pull toward the future.

In contrast to these divisions within time, the eternal has neither a beginning nor an end. "With the Lord one day is as a thousand years, and a thousand years as one day" (II Peter 3:8). Because it has neither dimensions nor limits, the eternal is often referred to as an eternal present—or an eternal now. When we are oriented to the present moment, therefore, we are open to the eternal's touch with time. It is the eternal now that gives time its qualitative dimension. We can recollect the eternal from the past and anticipate it for the future, but we can only know it in the present.

Paradoxically, death or one of its symbols may be the

catalyst for one's affirmation of life—for knowing its qualitative dimension. In mid-life my wife and I experienced what we never anticipated—the death of one of our children. It was sudden, tragic, and devastating. Through such pain, however, one gets a clearer perception of what is really important and what is not. The tragedy nudged us as a family to "let this moment count" in and of itself, rather than to treat it primarily as a preparation toward some future goal. To enjoy each other's presence in the family is sufficient justification for any moment of existence.

When we are future-oriented we miss much in the present moment that is more important for the quality of life than that for which we are striving. If you have experienced a death in the family, you know what I am describing. If you have not, I do not wish it for you, even if the experience does have a clarifying influence on one's values. I believe you can listen to God's Spirit in the midst of your blessings and perceive by faith the priorities of the moment that make for qualitative living.

When we are tomorrow-oriented we postpone enjoyment until the goals of tomorrow are achieved. This is far different from living in the present with hope for the future. Future orientation demotes the present to a subsidiary role. Although it appears to be the opposite, it is similar to waiting impatiently for "quitting time." In both situations the present is deprived of its distinctiveness. In contrast, living in the present in hope enriches the present because it is open-ended to the future. Though we focus on the present, we can also let it go, because we are moving in a purposeful direction.

It is important in mid-life to make this transition from future to present orientation if we have not done it previously, because to carry a future orientation into old age is to encounter a "time bomb." What happens to the future in old age in a culture that has no place for the aged? Deprived of opportunity by society and sometimes also by the aging process, older people may flipflop back to the past. They think and talk about the times when they were doing challenging things, when life was more interesting and when they were more important. Again the present is bypassed.

Older people living in the past are no more pathetic than middle-aged people living in the future. In remembering the good old days one is usually as unrealistic as when one looks to the future for satisfaction and fulfillment. In fact, there is probably more satisfaction in reliving the past. Since the past can be "touched up" by a selective memory so that it is actually not like it was, older people may get more satisfaction out of reliving the past than they did when they lived it.

Nostalgia brings meaning to the present only as a time to remember. It is the price one may pay in old age for not having lived in the present prior to becoming old. Although our society does not leave older people with much reason to live in the present, those who have experienced the *eternal now* will continue to experience it in old age. This does not excuse us from taking responsibility to change societal attitudes toward the elderly so that they *will* have a place in the societal mainstream. At the same time, we need to make positive investments in our own old age so that we take our meaning and purpose into it. Those who believe in the resurrection always have a future, and therefore always have a present. Because of this, every period in life is a golden age for the Christian—even mid-life!

5. Crisis in Meaning

Mid-life crises are essentially crises of meaning. Whatever gave sense to our lives before now is shaken. What's the use? we say when we reach our nadir. What's the purpose of it all? Why bother? Is it really worth the effort? Why go on? In each of these despairingly rhetorical questions the issue is clear—we have, temporarily at least, lost our sense of direction. The crisis this precipitates is painful. Our confidence sags under the weight of the despair, and we become painfully aware of our inadequacies.

AGE OF MELANCHOLY

So widespread is this mood of despair that our highest-ranking mental-health officer has described our age as "the age of melancholy." Dr. Gerald L. Klerman says melancholy is "our great social disease"—afflicting forty million Americans. A possible cause—"a gap between expectations and actuality" (reported in *Context,* June 1, 1979). Are we overstimulated in our affluent and permissive society to expect too much from life in a fallen world?

An interesting point about this epidemic of depression is

77

that it affects women from two to six times more often than men. Typical of these women is Kay who at forty-five was ready to give up. "I feel as if the bottom is dropping out of my life, and that I am nothing. I've promised to do too many things I don't care about for too many people that I don't really care about either. I am on all these committees and running like crazy, but it is all so stupid and meaningless. I want out—to quit trying—to be dead."

Why should such suffering afflict women more often than men in our society? The conclusion of many who have studied the matter is that the woman gives her highest priorities to pleasing others, which includes being attractive to, caring for, and being cared for by others. Instead of dealing directly with her own needs, she is more concerned about what others—particularly her family—want or need from her. This makes her dependent on others for her own self-esteem. Because of the changes in family relationships that take place in mid-life, depression may strike hardest at this time. If women risk more in loving than men do, they are more vulnerable to changes in their love relationships. Since these relationships have become less secure in our day, as marital and family ties are being increasingly severed, it is no coincidence that women would feel these ruptures with increased depression. (See "Depression," *Psychology Today*, April 1979.)

Another possible reason is that women tend to face their feelings more directly than men do and therefore are more conscious of emotional suffering. When men are depressed it is likely to be over their work, especially over problems that threaten their status in the competitive economic world. In dealing with these pressures men tend to turn to alcohol, since they have a significantly higher rate of alcoholism than women. Women, however, use three times as many prescription drugs, particularly tranquilizers, as men. The reason is obvious: women are more likely to go to a physician than men, more likely to be honest about their feelings with the physician than men, and therefore more likely to have tranquilizers and antidepressant drugs prescribed by their physicians than men.

Whether we look at depression among men or among women, the fact remains that there may be much to be depressed about. We have noted the stresses placed on family ties in this day of social change. In the realm of work, many of us are associated with the corporations and institutions that dominate the public sectors of our society. All institutions, including those associated with the church, have their stresses and strains. Whatever sort of institution we work for, it is not long before we become aware of the in-fighting, power struggles, unfair judgments and tactics, who's-in-with-whom and who's-out-to-get-whom that characterize the negative aspects of institutional life.

William Stringfellow compares these institutions to the "principalities and powers" mentioned in the Bible. He says they have their own distinct form of "fallenness," which is not simply the accumulated fallenness of the individuals that compose it. Instead, the institution's own distinct fallenness can corrupt these individuals and often does. Persons may participate in oppressive decisions and unjust actions as institutional people that they would reject as individuals. Stringfellow says that all institutions have a demonic potential, and only by maintaining checks and balances can this potential be curtailed.

Most of us in the work force probably agree with this description of institutional injustice. We are also quite sure that we give the institution within which we work more than we receive from it. At times we become disgruntled, feel unappreciated, convinced that our value to the institution is not really recognized. According to considerable research in this field, workers tend to follow a "self-serving bias" in their view of reality, seeing themselves in a more favorable light than they do their fellow employees. They regard their own views as less prejudiced than those of others with whom they work, even of their friends and neighbors. They also see themselves as more admirable and deserving. Persons in business, for example, perceive themselves as more ethical than the average business person. (See "How Christians Can Cope with Inflation: Getting off the 'Hedonic' Treadmill," by T.E. Ludwig and D.G. Myers, *The Christian Century,* May 30, 1979.) Reuel Howe describes a man with this self-serving bias in regard to his work. "When he thought of his job," says Howe, "he pictured himself as the only person on it who was active and responsible. He it was who had to think up all the questions and answers; only he could influence the issues and make the decisions" (Reuel Howe, *The Creative Years,* p. 25; Seabury Press, 1959). There have been times in my own work life when it seemed to me that I was the only one who could do the job the way it needed to be done.

The self-serving bias in our view of our role at work shows how subtly egotism distorts our perspective. This sort of self-exaltation is not the same as having a healthy self-image. Rather, it comes more under the apostle Paul's category of thinking of ourselves more highly than we ought to think

(Rom. 12:3). Basically, all such exaltation of ourselves over others is a compensation for a low self-image. The more healthy our self-image, the less comparatively we view others, and therefore the more open we are to receive what they have to offer in their own uniqueness. In contrast to our thinking more highly of ourselves than is warranted, a healthy self-image would lead us to "think with sober judgment," that is, with less bias and more objectivity, "according to the measure of faith which God has assigned" (Rom. 12:3). So the pains we experience from our work are due both to inherent disregard of human values on the part of institutions and corporations and to our own inherent egocentricity.

Stress on the job is an increasing form of suffering in our competitive environment and a major factor in undermining mental and physical health. Statistics speak "loud and clear" that if you want to live longer, you need to like your job. People in certain kinds of work tend to live longer than those in other kinds of work. On-the-job stress seems to be the important determining factor. A complementary influence is the degree of satisfaction one receives from the job. According to a study by Dr. Peter Brill, those in the professions have the highest job satisfactions—80 to 90 percent. White-collar workers are down to 50 percent and blue-collar workers to 10 to 20 percent. If you have a job in which the stress is undermining your satisfaction, there are a few things you can do about it, other than seeking another job. One is to work out a plan that will help you stay "on top of things." You may need to seek professional counsel in this regard. The least stressful jobs are those in which the worker feels most in control. A second thing is to put your energies into having a strong family life, for this may provide the support you need to endure stress positively. Thirdly, develop other interests than your job. Your work is not the same as your life. Diversify your interests; spread your energies. Rather than decreasing your work efficiency, such diversification of your interests may actually increase it, since some of the stress of the job is due to having invested too much of your ego in it.

I am sobered by the number of maturing families who are hurting or who have had their previous bouts with family pain. The more such people I know and the better I know them, the more I become involved in intercessory prayer for them. There is a wide range in these sufferings. Besides depression that may be attributed to fluctuations in our family life or in our job situation, there is the grief that some persons experience in the loss of a family relationship. Paul and Vera were away on a brief trip when their youngest child, a ten-year-old daughter, was stricken with a rare disease. Although they returned immediately, the child remained in a coma until she died a week later. Said the grief-stricken father: "Never in all my days could I ever have dreamed that we would have known such a loss as this one. Sue was a very special little girl. Vera and I find ourselves wondering when the nightmare will end, and when our grief will be easier. We have an immense feeling of lostness. We pray to God for the strength to make it through each day."

Claudia's suffering was far different. She had planned a family get-together. Her oldest son had recently married and her oldest daughter had secured her own apartment. She arranged a time with both of them and with her husband and two children still at home. By that morning Claudia was high with anticipation. She had meticulously planned the meal, taking into account each person's favorite food. At four o'clock, the disappointments began. The eldest son called to say that his wife "had a bug" and they felt it would be better if they didn't come. He would have called sooner, he said, but they were hoping she would feel better and that they could still come. By six o'clock Bill, her husband, had not yet arrived. When the younger children complained about their hunger, Claudia reluctantly decided to begin the meal without him. When he arrived twenty minutes later he was all apologies. There had been an emergency at the plant and no time to call her. He was preoccupied during the whole meal, rarely speaking. Jack, the youngest, picking up the tension at the table, complained that the meat didn't taste good, and he left it and the vegetables on his plate. When the meal was over, Claudia went to her bedroom and cried. It was all to have been so nice, and look how it turned out! There had been other similar incidents of late. In her aching soul Claudia felt that she was the only one who really cared about the family.

Phyllis' suffering was physical. In early mid-life she developed arthritis in her hip and knee. At first it was periodic but the last two years it had become chronic. Her physician believed that she was too young to have artificial joints, and yet other treatments were not working. The pain was getting to her spirit. She could force herself to get around for only so long, and then she would give up and withdraw to her bed. It was hard on her husband and her children as well. They missed her participation in their activities, and they could sense her depression. As different as are the causes for the suffering of Paul and Vera, Claudia, and Phyllis, each of their sufferings was severe enough to threaten their sense of meaning. Why should this happen to me? What's the purpose of it? Why go on? What does it all mean?

THE NECESSITY FOR MEANING

Psychiatrist Viktor Frankl has founded a school of psychotherapy based on the principle that human beings require a sense of meaning for their lives in order to function well or even to survive. A survivor of Hitler's concentration camps, Frankl observed among the sufferers of these camps that those who had a purpose for living were more likely to endure than those who had lost that purpose. It is difficult to conceive of more horrendous suffering than that inflicted in these camps. As the severity of pain increases, the meaning of life is accordingly threatened. What is going on that I should hurt—or be hurt—so badly? This is a religious question, since it relates directly to providence. Is life a conglomeration of chancy happenings or is there a thread of meaning that runs through these happenings?

The character of Job in the Old Testament is an example of a person in the throes of such a crisis. Job was in later mid-life when the crisis developed—"in my autumn days" (Job 29:4), as he put it. As so often happens, his crisis grew out of a clash between his anticipations and what was actually transpiring. He thought he would end his days as an old man in the tranquillity that had marked his life. "Then I thought, 'I shall die in my nest, and I shall multiply my days as the sand'" (29:18). Instead, his good fortune suddenly collapsed. His sufferings covered the range of human pain. His ten children were killed by a tornado, his financial empire collapsed, his social status plummeted, and his physical health failed. This pileup of pain created a religious crisis. Job considered himself to be faithful to God. Why, then, had he experienced such reverses? Had God turned against him? When his friends tried to defend God against this accusation, Job demanded, "If it is not he, who then is it?" (9:24). In other words, if God isn't directing the course of events, who is?

Job expressed his despair by regretting that he had ever lived. "Why didst thou bring me forth from the womb?" he cried. "Would that I had died before any eye had seen me" (10:18). In his anguish he had given up hope. "The waters wear away the stones; the torrents wash away the soil of the earth; so thou destroyest the hope of man" (14:19). Emotionally and spiritually he was burned out. "In truth I have no help in me, and any resource is driven from me" (6:13). What bothered Job more than anything else was the silence of God. "I cry to thee and thou dost not answer me" (30:20).

God Speaks Through Suffering

As Job discovered, God can speak through suffering. Suffering is inevitable in a life terminated by death and infiltrated by death's symbols. After the serious illness of his wife, a prominent churchman wrote: "We thus joined after three decades the company of those who walk through valleys and find that they have deep shadows. How long we were spared!"

Our faith centers in a God who suffers. Psychoanalyst Carl Jung says that God's answer to Job's protest was in his own identification with human suffering when he became one of us in Jesus Christ. The silence of God in our sufferings can be deafening; his absence overwhelming. Lord, where are you?

At these times God is hidden behind the events that seem to deny his presence. He was hidden in the cross of Christ which at the time seemed to mock any semblance of providence. Jesus, as did Job, felt abandoned rather than supported. "My God, my God, why hast thou forsaken me?" As Paul Tillich has pointed out, Jesus showed his absolute faith when he then said, "Father, into thy hands I commit my spirit." He committed himself to the God whom he felt had abandoned him, trusting that he was not really absent, but only hidden behind the tragic events of time.

To span the gap between anticipation and actuality that seems to be the aggravant of so much pain in mid-life, we need to become clear concerning what God has promised and what he has not promised. God has not promised to spare us from the symptoms and symbols of death. Our faith does not make us immune to the diseases and failures and tragedies that affect human life. What God has promised is that he will be present with us in all our ways—that he will give us the strength to endure whatever adversities we encounter. He has further promised to utilize all our experiences as means toward our own fulfillment—fulfillment of our calling. In other words, he has promised to put it all together—to supply meaning to our lives in the midst of our sufferings—and to integrate us around the hope for healing and overcoming.

Pain itself may be "saying" something to us. Physical pain often reprimands us for abusing our bodies, or urges us to care for them. The same is true with mental pain. It may be saying something to us about our way of life, our values, our attitude toward ourselves and others. We need to be sensitive to what our pains are saying.

Suffering has different effects on different persons. Intense pain demands our full attention. When it is chronic, it absorbs most of our energies, turning us in on ourselves. Suffering can also be a means for personal growth. One's compassion for others in their sufferings is enhanced when one knows what it is like to suffer. It was the compassion of Jesus that drew him to "the poor and maimed and blind and lame" (Luke 14:21). Referring to the people of the church as members of the body of Christ, the apostle Paul says, "If one member suffers, all suffer together; if one member is honored, all rejoice together" (I Cor. 12:26). Our sufferings can identify us more closely with the human family through the empathy that comes from knowing our own pain.

In our own family, however, suffering may move us to *over*-empathize. We do not want our children to go through the pain that we have experienced. Yet if we try to spare them, we may deprive them of the experiences they need as preparation for life in this world. Rudolf Dreikurs, an authority in family living, says that parents need to allow their children to experience the natural consequences of their own actions, even when painful, so they can learn from the experience. In this way, he says, they develop into responsible persons who cope realistically with life. While they need our help in dealing with their challenges, they need also to *own* their own problems, and to be responsible for resolving them. If we realize that our sufferings, besides being painful, were also instrumental in our development toward maturity, we can temper our empathy for our children in their pains so that it provides the support they need to take responsible action rather than to become an obstacle to this action.

CRISIS IN PROVIDENCE

In a crisis of meaning we search for a divine purpose. As Frankl says, if we can figure out why things are happening the way they are, we can live with them better. Sometimes we come up with strange conclusions, since it is easier to live with a strange conclusion than with no conclusion. A friend of Paul and Vera's tried to explain why their child had died. "God was probably taking her now to spare her some greater suffering in the future," she said. They did not find much comfort in this. It is hard to live without answers, particularly if our faith seems to depend on them.

Sometimes our crises require decisions from us that we feel inadequate to make. What should I do? If only I knew what God's will is! Sensing God's direction for us in any particular moment may depend on a great deal of prayer and meditation, consultation with others, and personal counseling. But there are some things that we know about God's ways that give us a general direction in which to move. This direction centers in the values and priorities of the Kingdom of God as taught and lived by Jesus, values that enhance the quality of human living. An obvious place to begin, therefore, is to make decisions that reflect a priority for persons over money, property, and other things. Material things need to take second place to our relationships with persons. If a child accidently breaks something costly that we treasure, how do we react? Things are important, broken things

are to be regretted—but they are less important than the one who broke them. Therefore, our reaction should not reject the person responsible. Damage to things is lamentable, but it is not the ultimate loss.

Is there anything within reason that the breaker can do to restore that which is broken? Let reparations be made as an act of responsibility, but not as a punishment. Is there something one can learn from the incident that would help in future situations? These are areas of exploration for some positive meaning to an otherwise negative experience.

Our relationships are also more important than our pride. Our children, or spouse, may do things that embarrass us. How do you tell your friends that your daughter is living with a man to whom she is not married—without feeling a loss of self-esteem? How do you cope with the rage you feel in knowing that your spouse has been unfaithful even though the affair is over? When our pride is wounded, we want to retaliate against the offender or at least to withdraw from him or her, rather than to take the initiative for reconciliation. Knowing that we ourselves live in a covenant of forgiveness with God helps us to put relationships before our pride, as we extend this forgiveness to those who have hurt us. When we keep open the doors to our relationships, we are also keeping open the possibility for change.

One of the ironies in family living is that affection which is potentially abundant in families tends to be severely rationed. Why should this be? Philip Slater says that we keep affection scarce so that we can put more of our energies into our work and thereby acquire more cultural symbols of our worth. The bumper sticker, "Have you hugged your child today?" is on the right track. God made us not merely as souls but also as bodies, and we receive love also through our bodies. So don't ration your hugs and tender touches. We all need them.

There is no surer way to discontent than to seek first the status symbols of a nice house, a new car, a higher salary, and membership in the right clubs. All these things may be good in themselves and thus desirable, but the importance with which we invest them gives them the power to deprive us of contentment. Acquisitiveness has its own built-in sabotage of quality living. Psychologists Thomas E. Ludwig and David G. Myers describe two principles from psychological research that explain our apparent predisposition to discontent. The first is the *adaptation-level phenomenon*. According to this principle we determine our satisfaction or dissatisfaction on the basis of our prior experience. It is something *more* than we have had that makes us satisfied—something *less* makes us dissatisfied. However, after we have lived with the changed situation for a while, whether it is positive or negative, we adapt to it and it becomes neutral. Only something in addition to wht we have at the present can then give pleasure. In a recent survey nearly half of those who said they were satisfied with their present standard of living also said that the absence of further increases would be disappointing or even disturbing. Only more and more, then, can keep us content. This is probably why striving for more becomes an end in itself, since the *more*, when attained, provides only a short-lived satisfaction. Barbara Jordan, in explaining her surprising decision not to seek reelection to the House of Representatives, put it well. "Getting there," she said, "is more fun than being there. It has always been this way with me."

The other principle is the *relative-deprivation principle.* This principle is based on the tendency to compare ourselves with others, and especially *significant* others. We compare ourselves only with those who have more than we and not with those who have less. Consequently most of us are dissatisfied with our socioeconomic situation because there are others who are doing better. There seems to be no end to these rising aspirations that leave us forever discontented. We are back again on the treadmill for an illusionary contentment.

In contrast to the acquisitive route to happiness, the writer of I Timothy says, "There is great gain in godliness with contentment; for we brought nothing into the world, and we cannot take anything out of the world; but if we have food and clothing, with these we shall be content" (I Tim. 6:6–8). Ecclesiastes comes to the same conclusion: "Then I saw that all toil and all skill in work come from a man's envy of his neighbor. This also is vanity and a striving after wind" (Eccl. 4:4). Ludwig and Myers also come to the same conclusion: "Simple living unclutters the heart and makes room for those things that have ultimate value" (Ludwig and Myers, "How Christians Can Cope with Inflation," p. 610).

When the Scripture writer says that godliness with contentment is great gain, he is not only describing the source of those "things that have ultimate value" but is also showing us another place to begin in regard to God's will. God calls us to take our devotion to him with us into our crises, so that he can provide the security and the hope we need to endure the crises. In other words, God calls us to trust him. The most difficult time to trust God is when we are experiencing a crisis; yet it is precisely at such a time that we most need this trust, and it is to such a time that trust is most applicable.

When things are going well we receive a lot of support for our sense of meaning from what is happening in our midst. In crisis moments this support is largely removed. Faith in God, however, can provide us with "the evidence of things not seen" (Heb. 11:1, KJV). Unfortunately at such times we tend to distrust this "evidence" and desire instead evidence we can see. Trusting begins when we face our resistance to trust and choose to take the leap of faith. It is the Spirit of God who is calling us to make this leap, and our choice is really our response to his overture.

As a pastoral counselor I have at times challenged a coun- selee by saying, "Now is the time for your faith to affirm itself." I have said this to myself also when I needed to hear it. I am not spared stress because I work for a theological seminary. Seminaries, seminary teachers, and seminary stu- dents are *in* the world and also *of* it. So I have said to myself, "Now is the time for you to trust rather than to become preoccupied with negative feelings." I don't find this any easier than you do. In fact, to trust God in moments of stress is about the most difficult thing I do. Everything within me and outside of me seems to conspire against it. At the same time I find that trusting in God is also the easiest thing I do, since I need simply to respond to his invitation to cast my cares on him—to let him have them. Once I do this, he seems to "take over," supplying me with the peace that passes understanding, at least intermittently.

BELIEF IN PROVIDENCE

Our capacity to trust is directly related to our belief in providence. The British psychoanalyst Ernest Jones said, "What one really wants to know about the divine purpose is its intentions toward oneself." The good news of Christ is that God's intentions toward us are *good*. "He who did not spare his own Son but gave him up for us all, will he not also give us all things with him?" (Rom. 8:32). The cross of Christ is God's sign that he is *for* us. "If God is for us, who is against us?" (Rom. 8:31).

Once we believe that God is for us—that his intentions toward us are good—we are ready to receive what God can give us in any current crisis or moment of pain. When Job insisted that God did not answer his cries for help, Elihu wisely responded, "God speaks in one way, and in two, though man does not perceive it" (Job 33:14). Elihu's insight gave Job a different perspective on the silence of God: it may more accurately be termed the deafness of man. Job had his own particular idea of how God would answer him. When he didn't perceive this answer, he concluded that God had not spoken. Elihu believed Job's evidence to be insufficient. God may be speaking in a way we do not anticipate and consequently we may miss what he is saying. Elihu, in effect, told Job to look around, to cock his ears in a different direction.

When we choose to trust God to get us through a crisis, by this very act we project meaning into the crisis. Since trust is actually our response to God's promise to help us, it provides the hope we need. When we thus perceive the hidden God, the ears and eyes of faith offer us a fuller perspective within which to view our situation. Our trust is called a leap of faith because by it we "leap over" what otherwise appear to be insuperable barriers. The most these barriers can do to God's guidance is to pose a detour in the route. He can even make profitable use of the detour.

Faith in providence is itself a source of good news, making possible a joy that is not dependent, at least totally, on what happens *to* us. The joy of the Lord can remain when the usual reasons for happiness are not there. Our relationship with God can continue relatively stable through faith when other props that normally we depend on are not available. When we trust in God in the midst of our crises, we will find it easier also to trust others—our spouse, our children. Therefore, we may be less demanding in our desire for their support. The trust we place in them is a positive influence in their own development. Most of us thrive on the trust that others, particularly significant others, have in us.

6. Freedom to Grow

God can use our crises in mid-life for our personal growth as we move to the next stage of our life—and the life of our family. We are free to leave the past and to look toward the future with hope. We are in passage, but the movement is neither steady nor smooth. Unlike bodily growth which is linear, spiritual growth is best described by the Biblical figure of dying and rising. We die to the old and rise to the new. The figure, of course, comes from Christ's death and resurrection. Baptism is our identification with Christ in which we are "buried with him by baptism into death." Our old egocentric self is crucified with Christ, and as Christ was raised from the dead, so also we rise to a new life which is open and receptive. Personal growth is a series of ups and downs, with each down providing the possibility for a new beginning—another resurrection. This is why Paul Tournier can say that there is no such thing as a stable Christian life. The old resists dying—and new beginnings are characterized by "labor and travail."

Though the way of personal growth is wrenching and

95

upheaving, the direction is clear. As those baptized into Christ, we grow into his likeness. He is a model for human maturity, the human being God intended us to be. So we are to "grow up in every way into him," into "the measure of the stature of the fulness of Christ" (Eph. 4:13, 15).

The freedom we have for change is the freedom to change ourselves and not others. Perhaps this is disappointing. We are concerned about our children, our spouse, our parents, and want so much to see change take place in their lives. Prayers for this change are influential. Changes in your own life are also a factor. Elton and Pauline Trueblood wrote a statement that made a strong impression on me as a young parent.

> The parent makes the mistake, frequently, of concentrating on the child, when he would help the child more if he would concentrate upon himself. The parent must guard, accordingly, against the danger of too much self-sacrifice. If the sacrifice is obvious it defeats its purpose. Much as we help those whom we love by performing services for them, we help them more by being composed and happy persons. More good is done in personal relations by the habit of happiness than by obvious deeds of kindness. (D.E. Trueblood and P.C.G. Trueblood, *Recovery of Family Life,* pp. 93–94; Harper & Brothers, 1953)

As I look back on that impression I believe it was an abstract appreciation for a good insight rather than anything I seriously applied to my life. Over the years, there were events that nudged me into seriously applying it. As a result I have even a greater appreciation for the Truebloods' statement. I believe that whatever time, energy, and interest you put into your own personal growth will have its good influence on the family, even though it may not be apparent at the moment.

The basis for personal growth is the freedom to face reality and remain positive. Depression is an example of facing reality and remaining negative. Denial is an example of remaining positive at the expense of facing reality. The means for the freedom to be both realistic and positive is God's covenant of forgiveness that is shared with us through baptism. By drawing a curtain on the past, his forgiveness makes it possible to look at the present without the distortions from the past. Emancipated from these negative holdovers, we can envision the future in hope.

God's covenant of forgiveness applies directly to our family relationships. Who of us is not painfully aware of errors in judgment, in value choices, mishandled emotions, falling into old and discredited patterns of behavior, of being one-sided in our perceptions? Parenthood is a highly responsible task, and most of us enter into it with little awareness of what it entails. We have some definite ideas about improving on our own parents, but that is about it. When our good intentions yield not-so-good results, we tend to blame ourselves. In its frustration over problems of young people, society blames the parents, and this only reinforces our guilt. If it did any good just to feel guilty, there might be some redeeming features to this heavy burden, but our guilt feelings are more likely to be an additional obstacle to our parental competence. Until we are reconciled with ourselves in our guilt, we have no freedom to grow—to change.

Some of our parental guilt may be exaggerated, but whether exaggerated or justified, the purpose of guilt is to effect changes in behavior. The way to accomplish this purpose is to resolve our guilt through reconciliation. When we are forgiven, we need not deny the negative to be positive. Instead, we can look at the negative—specifically our sins and shortcomings as parents—in the context of God's unconditional acceptance.

Forgiveness helps us also to accept our anger. Some of us are carrying a load of anger in addition to guilt, though we may contain it most of the time. When it breaks out, however, we overstate the case, to put it mildly. Even when we contain our anger, it slips out indirectly. We "innocently" dig people, or resist their suggestions, or withdraw from them. God knows when we are angry and still loves us. So it is best to acknowledge our anger at least to ourselves and to God. Then we can seek in a constructive way to deal with it: perhaps by acknowledging it also to our family by simply saying "I'm angry!" as Parent Effectiveness Training teaches us; perhaps by retreating to the bathroom until we calm down, as Dreikurs advises us; perhaps also by "letting it out" to God in prayer, as the psalmists often did.

Our faith is not in forgiveness but in the forgiveness of *God.* As the hymn says, "God is the ruler yet." In our guilt it seems that our errors and sins are the rulers. There is some egotism in this position. As one mother expressed it, "My self-image is so low that anything that goes wrong is my fault." Some of us are "guilt collectors." Others are "anxiety collectors," which is simply the other side of the coin. Although in a negative dimension, we exaggerate our own importance. If we believe that God is bigger than our blunders and not immobilized by our sins, we are emancipated from the egotism that tends to fix us in guilt and anxiety. We are not the ultimate influence in our children's lives; our faith in God adds another dimension to what we see and hear.

Life-Style Consonant with Our Faith

Christian families may talk better about a life-style consonant with their faith than they live it. Children, then, receive double signals. Since they are not so heavily invested in the world as their parents, they can be critical of the "hypocrisy" of their elders. They are often more concerned than their parents about the "present distress" (I Cor. 7:26) of our planet. They are concerned about the depletion of our natural resources. They realize that we are the energy gluttons of the globe and are willing to face up to it. In the early days of the gasoline shortage a Michigan congressman argued against a tax on gas-guzzling cars by saying that some people need large cars to pull their boats and trailers. It may be difficult now to comprehend such parochial reasoning. Those who take their Christian vocation seriously know that they must be concerned about more than their own immediate circle of acquaintances. John Wesley said the world was his parish. The whole human family is our concern. What America needs is people who model a voluntary simplification of their life-style because of the "present distress."

Such modeling is needed for the good of the country as well as the planet. Yet you can no more expect a self-indulged people to respond favorably to your example of a simplified life-style than you can expect the institutions that employ you to applaud when you affirm your concern for honesty, justice, and compassion at your job. The rejection you may receive is what is meant by "taking up your cross," an obligation laid upon us when we identify with Christ. "If any man would come after me, let him deny himself and take up his cross and follow me" (Mark 8:34). The cross is a symbolic term for whatever "flack" we receive when we are faithful to the concerns of our calling. Christ's cross— a literal one—which he could have avoided was accepted by him as the inevitable consequence of his calling.

Sometimes I think we are so indoctrinated in the knowledge of how God used Christ's cross for our redemption that we forget about the sociological forces that placed him on that cross. When I asked a student why Jesus was crucified, he answered, "So that God could redeem us through it." "That is a theological interpretation of the event," I said, "but what was the historical occasion?" When he seemed perplexed by the question I reminded him of what he obviously knew but which did not seem relevant at the moment. Christ was crucified because as a prophet he exposed the injustice and hypocrisy of his society. The truth was so threatening to those in control that they agreed that one man should die rather than the whole nation be torn apart. It was this way also before Christ—the prophets of Israel were usually persecuted—and it has been this way since. You may not be killed in America, but you may be ignored or criticized or even fired.

But the other side of the coin is that your concern for justice and truth and compassion for the oppressed leads you to the joy of Christ. The whole nation would not have perished if the people had listened to Jesus, but it would have changed. Many of us are like the farmer with the bumper crop in Jesus' parable, who could think of nothing better to do with his surplus than to build bigger barns in which to store it. If someone had suggested that he share it with others, he probably would have considered this threatening to his own security. Actually it would have fostered his security. No wonder God called him a fool. Even regarding his own welfare, this is precisely what he was. In desiring to hold on to everything, he lost everything.

Jesus' teaching was the opposite. "For whoever would save his life will lose it; and whoever loses his life for my sake and the gospel's will save it" (Mark 8:35). This is the way of wisdom, and America needs people who will adopt this model.

Utilizing the Resources of the Church

Our growth into Christ's stature is a corporate process as well as an individual one. The body of believers of which he is the head is composed of many interrelated members. Jesus stressed this corporate dimension of his following by saying, "For where two or three are gathered in my name, there am I in the midst of them" (Matt. 18:20). Our faith is not simply a matter between ourselves and God, but also of the people of God with God.

The people of God are subject to much criticism, some of which justified and some not. Because the people of God are highly visible in local congregations and in denominational and interdenominational church organizations, they are also highly vulnerable. More in terms of ethical conduct and compassionate behavior is expected from a church group than from a fraternal organization. The charge of hypocrites in the church is a frequent blast rarely leveled at other institutions. The implication is that believers in Christ are committed to the highest behavioral standards, and any departure from these disqualifies them from creditability as the people of God. I asked a friend why he did not affiliate with a church since he was reared as a Christian and considered himself a believer. His answer was that he did not believe that he lived up to the behavioral standards that such affiliation required. Obviously the people of God are not confined to those whose names are on church rolls. At the same time, those who belong to the churches have publicly committed themselves to the corporate dimension of their faith in a most visible way.

The church is a human institution, "in the world but not of it," and yet subject to all the institutional temptations that come from the world. Perhaps you are critical of your own congregation or your denomination, and for good reason. Sometimes it seems we find more resistance than support from our church for concerns for justice and compassion. The church's history in these matters has been spotty. Racial prejudice is as rampant in some churches as in the communities surrounding them. Local congregations can be self-serving rather than self-giving, with little awareness of their responsibility to the total community in which they are located, let alone their global responsibilities.

Obviously if the church is to be justified, it is justified only by the grace of God and not by its own works. But this is the way that families and individuals are also justified. So you as an individual believer and your family as a Christian family have a lot in common with your congregation. Prior to the celebration of Holy Communion, a member informed his pastor that he felt unworthy to commune. "Then you should join us," said the pastor. "It is *for* sinners."

The body of believers in your parish—with all of its petty bickering and insensitivity to human need—is your family's extended family. Your congregation may need your forgiveness as well as your witness, but your family also needs your congregation. This gathering of individuals and families in Christ's name offers us the larger family that we all need for our development. Individual families turned in on themselves suffer the same distorting effects as do individuals who turn in on themselves. Parents need other adults to share with them in their parental responsibility. When I was in my teens an important adult in my life was my Sunday school teacher, who was also my scoutmaster in the Boy Scout troop sponsored by my church. He was a supplement to my own parents. He lost his only child in a sudden illness and the youths in the Sunday school class and in the Scout troop helped him to survive. Perhaps because of this experience I have always been pleased when other adults took a personal interest in my children.

The congregation is the family of God in which individual families support each other. The baptism of children before the assembled congregation is not only a baptism into Christ but also a baptism into Christ's body, the church. The rite symbolizes the child's inclusion in the family of God. The church is a *worshiping* community in which those gathered in Christ's name participate in an act of devotion that removes the ambiguity over who is God. As creatures we join together to acknowledge the presence of the Creator in whose image we are created.

The church is also a *witnessing* community, having a purpose that goes beyond its own self-serving, the mission of Christ to the world. We need such a purpose, as do our families, for our growth and development. We need to be integrated around a purpose bigger than ourselves—bigger than our families. Youths are especially sensitive to this need. In their natural idealism they desire to devote their lives to something more than to the accumulation of our society's status symbols. This is one reason they are drawn to the religious cults that have been the notorious Pied Pipers of recent times. The tune they play draws our children because it calls them to a higher cause. Granted that some of these cults have been repeatedly exposed as exploiters of youthful idealism, the fact that their charismatic leaders offer their followers the security of an extended family and an idealistic purpose to which to dedicate themselves is tempting to those who are lonely and lack a vision.

Because a youth joins a cult does not automatically mean that his or her local church was not offering a challenge. It does mean that for one reason or another the youth did not hear this challenge as an answer to his or her need. It is also possible that the church did not reach out to the youth as did the cult. In that case you along with others in the church should confer about how your church's mission can be made more concrete in today's world, so that youths as well as others can be challenged to devote themselves to it. As an activity of the extended family, this conferring should include some of these youths. So long as the people of a congregation refer to their church as *we*, they will utilize their energies to improve the ministry of the congregation. When they begin to refer to it as *they*, the same energies will be used to criticize the congregation for its shortcomings and failures.

We need each other in order to receive the freedom to

grow. The word in the Christian tradition for this mutual assistance is *ministry*. Unfortunately, the word has become so identified with the clergy that its meaning for lay persons is diminished. The *minister* ministers, but so should the rest of God's people. We are all ministers one to another in the body of Christ. This mutual ministry not only helps each of us and our families to grow but also contributes to the effectiveness of the congregation as a family. In "speaking the truth in love," we upbuild each other as well as the congregation. Obviously members of the extended family will differ on many things, as do members of the smaller families. The important distinction is that we differ with *respect*. Our relationship is more important than our uniformity; our unity is "rooted and grounded in love" (Eph. 3:17).

7. Respect for Self, Spouse, and Children

Any crisis that draws us closer to God and to the priorities of his Kingdom will have its good effect also on our other relationships. One good effect is the way we approach others, namely, with increased respect. Respect entails courtesy, humility, and genuine interest. In contrast to honor, it refers to an attitude toward one's equals. We will concentrate on respect as it pertains to our family relationships.

BEGIN WITH SELF

The first of these family relationships is our relationship to ourself. This is a good place to begin because the way in which we relate to ourselves serves as a model for the way in which we relate to others in the family. It is important, therefore, that we cultivate our own company. "We need to listen," says Henri Nouwen, "to our own inner voices." We can easily bypass these voices in our concern for relating to God and to other people. If we do, however, we will actually hinder these relationships. The neglected voices within are projected into our other "listenings," with the result that we hear distortedly. Self-respect follows the old law that Jesus reemphasized: "You shall love your neighbor as yourself." In Ephesians this law is applied to marriage: "Let each one of you love his wife as himself" (Eph. 5:33). Since our love for ourselves is the model for our other loves, we need to give it attention.

Respect is an attribute of love. Paul describes it in his well-known I Corinthians, ch. 13, particularly vs. 4 to 8. "Love is patient and kind; love is not jealous or boastful; it is not arrogant or rude. Love does not insist on its own way; it is not irritable or resentful; it does not rejoice at wrong, but rejoices in the right. Love bears all things, believes all things, hopes all things, endures all things. Love never ends."

These descriptions of love's behavior are also descriptions of respect. Love—respect—is "patient and kind." Some people defend their demanding ways by saying that they are no harder on others than they are on themselves. While they are correct in their awareness of the model, they could change the way they are modeling. If we are patient and kind with ourselves, we will be no less patient and kind with others.

Showing respect for ourselves means doing what is beneficial for our total person, physically, mentally, spiritually. These dimensions of our being are interrelated, mutually affecting one another. Respect toward ourselves would limit the self-destructiveness that seems to characterize the way many people live, perhaps including those who are "hard on themselves." They lack respect for themselves as persons and seek to compensate in some other way, particularly through their achievements.

Our bodies seem to take the biggest beating in our disrespect for ourselves. Disregard for the body is sometimes encouraged by religious teachings that implicitly downgrade the physical side of life. We need to restore our bodies to their Biblical significance, to their status as the "temple of the Holy Spirit within you" (I Cor. 6:19). In respecting our bodies we need to be concerned about what we eat. In a land richly blessed with food, Americans are often malnourished because they are conditioned by a bombardment of advertisement to prefer foods that are low in nutrition. Our penchant for sugary drinks and desserts, processed and refined foods, and the fast-food menus is taking its toll on our health in mid-life and especially in our later years. Unfortunately these foods are becoming a symbol of the American way of life. Fast-food sales in 1978 totaled $21,000,000,000, a 17 percent increase over 1977. The number of fast-food establishments is estimated at 66,000, an increase of 14,000 in the last two years. The problem is not just in the high fat and low nutrition of the food but also in the waste and pollution of these establishments. To supply only one of these, namely, McDonald's, with their throwaway paper for one year requires approximately 630 square miles of forest *(Nutrition Action,* June 1979, p. 10). As a caricature of our "affluent poverty," two of our wealthiest people, Howard Hughes and Barbara Hutton, died not only friendless but of illnesses related directly to malnutrition. Hughes reportedly lived mostly on ice cream and Hutton on soft drinks.

In mid-life your body may not take the abuse it did in your earlier days. Read the labels on the food you buy to see what you are actually receiving. Commercial cereals, for example, often list sugar as the second largest ingredient. Salt is another frequent ingredient as well as chemical additives for preservation, coloring, and the like. You did not contract to buy all of these when you bought the cereal, but you get them regardless. The same is true with most of the other processed foods. It is not easy to protect your body by what you eat, but it can be done.

We show respect for our bodies also by how we use them. Technological advances have turned us into a sedentary people. We are addicted to the automobile for our mobility and prefer to watch the professionals rather than to play ourselves. The gasoline shortage is good for our bodies, because it is an inducement to walk and to bicycle. The large increase in the number of people of all ages who are running, bicycling, swimming, hiking, and pursuing other forms of exercise that stimulates the cardiovascular system is one of the most positive changes to occur in recent times. If you are not already doing so, start running. Since we all ran as children, it is an activity we don't have to "learn." I began to run about ten years ago and thoroughly enjoy it. Have a physical examination first to see if there is any reason why you should not run. Begin slowly—fifty yards, a hundred yards, a quarter of a mile—and add a few yards each time. Run every other day to give your muscles their needed rest. Think in terms of years, rather than weeks, as you build up to a mile, to two miles, three miles. Run leisurely; enjoyment and not speed is the prior goal. Running has its good effect also on the mind and the spirit. Those who run regularly do not need chemical stimulants to "feel good." If running is out of the question for you, consider walking or swimming. A brisk daily walk may do as much for your constitution as running, and swimming is an excellent exercise for bones, joints, and muscles.

Your mind also needs to be nourished. Respect for it means to develop its potential for interest and knowledge. The overused cliché, "food for thought," is still an apt metaphor. Our mind needs exercise in both its thinking and feeling capacities. The parochial scope of so many people's interests limits their consciousness, inhibits their intellectual development, and predisposes them to negative feelings. When this stifling of mental capacities takes place in mid-life, the prognosis for the quality of life in old age is exceedingly dim.

The mental stimulation that is most satisfying comes from an involvement with people. Knowledge that includes wisdom is directly related to knowing people. Curiosity is the stimulus for knowledge. It moves us to search for understanding, to draw others out in their particular insights. Each of us is a potential teacher of the other.

Reading is another source of mental nourishment. *The Christian Century* for a lengthy period listed the books that specific persons said had shaped their lives. Although the lists varied widely, there was a core of classics that were continually repeated. These are examples of books that stretch our minds and "make us think." You can add to the stimulation of your reading by organizing a reading group of interested persons that meets regularly to discuss a selected book. The Bible has been the source of much stimulation for Christians through the centuries. Since God reveals himself through the Word, the study of the Bible brings knowing God and knowledge of God together in a devotional experience.

Writing is another discipline that stimulates our minds. It helps us to clarify and formulate our thoughts, as we search for the right word to express the shade of meaning that we have in mind. Keep a journal in which you record your reflections and insights. Besides the stimulation of writing it, a journal helps us to remember what we have learned so that we can build on these insights.

The dimension of our person that reaches out to God, our spirit, needs care as does our body and mind. This care likewise consists in proper nourishment and exercise. We provide our spirit both when we allocate a regular time to *center* ourselves, to focus on the values and priorities that give meaning to our lives. As we center ourselves on a disciplined basis we will discover that meditation and prayer will occur naturally other times during the day. The situation is similar to what Marriage Encounter couples discover when they take time for daily dialogue. As one husband said: "Before we began our dialoguing I rarely thought of my wife and family while at work. I suppose it was because my work is very demanding. Since we have been dialoguing, however, I noticed that I frequently think of her and the family while at work."

The similarity of this observation to the effects of prayer and meditation on our spirit could be anticipated, since in both Testaments our relationship to God is compared to a marriage. Dialogue with God is not only good for our spirit; this experience has good effects also on our mind and body.

In showing respect for ourselves physically, mentally, and spiritually, we model this respect for our children. They may resist the model at the moment, poke fun at it, or even attack it, but the chances are good that later they will appreciate it. Ralph Nader's diligence in study grew out of his family experience at the supper table. Besides eating, the family talked. Each person was expected to say what he or she thought concerning the subject. Nader's father presided over the sessions and they often lasted three or four hours. This and other examples ought to encourage us to trust that our children will recognize at some time whatever wisdom is involved in our parental modeling.

RESPECT FOR SPOUSE

At the close of the longest passage on marriage in the New Testament are the words: "Let the wife see that she respects her husband" (Eph. 5:33). The Greek word translated "to respect" actually means "to reverence." One might see in this word a reflection of first-century society's male dominance. Yet reverence for another person does not necessarily indicate his or her superiority. Although reverence is directed ultimately to God, it is by implication directed also toward his creation, as Albert Schweitzer taught a "reverence for life." There is also a proper reverence for those created in God's image. The attitude is similar to the respect that a husband would give to his wife if he "loved her as himself" (Eph. 5:33).

While respect for persons should characterize all our relationships, it is particularly important in marriage where two people are joined in an intimacy that is uniquely described as "one flesh." Without mutual respect this intimacy can change into hatred.

The renegotiation of the marital contract to which we previously referred is really renegotiating the meaning of mutual respect in a marriage at mid-life. While the contract would vary according to the individual marriage, respect for our spouse focuses on a few basic aspects of marriage. First, the companionship dimension of marriage should be renewed, if need be. Respect is to see our spouse as a person and not as a role or function, and as a *unique* person, with fascinating and distinctive characteristics. This respect is the basis for enjoying the other's presence and the motivation to do enjoyable things together.

Secondly, respect for the other means that we work at improving our stimulus into what is so obviously a stimulus-response relationship. If we are in doubt concerning the specifics of this stimulus improvement, a little dialogue with our spouse should reveal them.

Thirdly, respect for the other means that we accept irritations in our relationship as a concomitant of intimacy rather than as justifiable reasons for criticism. When our perfectionist tendencies lead us to take these irritations too seriously and thereby to lose our sense of humor, we are more than likely to become "arrogant and rude."

Finally, respect for our spouse means that we make a serious attempt in mid-life to sort out the old tapes that have been accumulated through the years and that are obstructing new beginnings in the relationship. As the novelist Balzac said, "Marriage must constantly conquer the monster that devours, its name is habit." Mid-life is the time to try new things in your marriage, to overcome resistance to change—"to believe all things and hope all things." It is possible that your marital relationship also may become a new creation.

Since marriage is a partnership, you may find it helpful to talk about your marital growth together. Hear each other out. The common family complaint is that members do not listen to one another. I hear it from *my* family, and I am working on it. Listening to another is perhaps the number one mark of respect. Talking together about your marital possibilities may stimulate ideas that neither of you would arrive at by yourselves. If such ideas are mutually owned, you are both more likely to act on them. In addition, talking together is itself a practice in intimacy and therefore good for your marriage. "Talk," says Caroline Bird, "is the most important aphrodisiac."

We must invest time, energy, and initiative into our marriage so that it will continue, though the children of our marriage may leave. In open dialogue on sensitive issues, you may discover yourself becoming defensive. If you are like most of us, you can expect it. Our defensiveness usually highlights the areas where we ourselves feel vulnerable and unacceptable. Once we are willing to accept this, we have resources in our faith to cope with our defensiveness.

RESPECT FOR OUR CHILDREN

Respect for our children means respect for their individuality and particularly for their *space*. It is a temptation to parents to invade their children's space because it seems to be the quickest way to control them. Respect would mean trusting them instead—and trusting God who also is their Parent. It may help us to develop this respect if we recognize what family counselors call "family systems." You have a distinct kind of relationship with each of your children as does your spouse, and they also with you. What goes on in this relationship as well as in the constellation of all the family relationships is described as a system. There is sufficient repetition in these goings-on for us to recognize the system. Thus in any particular transaction in a particular relationship both you and the child contribute something characteristic to the system. Once we know what our contribution is, we can evaluate whether or not it is a manifestation of respect.

For example, in families where one member has become dependent on drugs, the others are described as potential co-dependents. This does not mean that they are also chemically dependent, but rather that they are so affected by the other's dependency that they are controlled by it. This shows up in the way they relate to that person. Co-dependency exists with other family problems as well. The troubled person easily becomes the focus of that family's concern or anxiety, and in this regard the family scapegoat. Family counselors have discovered that it is better to counsel with the whole family than just with the troubled member, since the co-dependents also need help if the family systems are to change for the better.

As with other pains, we need to ask ourselves what the family pain is doing *to* us and *for* us. Since family systems are complex, raising this question may help family members to investigate their contribution to family problems or at least to the continuation of them.

While it is true that parents need to share the burdens of their children, it is also true that each child must bear his or her own burden. Respect for the child means, among other things, permitting the child to do this. Having parents that "go through the valley" with them is important to resolving their problems. Those same parents, however, need to respect the boundary between the responsibility of the child and their own responsibilities. Respect for the child means respect for the child's capacity to handle his or her own problems, provided needed support is given. We can and should "go through the valley" *with* them, but not *for* them. In giving them our respect we are giving them permission to grow into their own identity—to bear their own pains.

Systems change and need to change with the growing maturity of the child. Here as elsewhere we parents need to let go of the past and enter into the new. I recently talked to a mid-life father who said he was feeling so much better in all ways because he was finally able to let his children lead their own lives. Respecting our children helps us to let go of them in their readiness to venture out, and yet to maintain the open door for their needed returns. This flexibility within the system prevents us from the arbitrariness of our own preconceived notions—from "insisting on our own way." Respect within the system leaves room for dialogue in the decision-making process.

With this insight into love as respect, we bring our involvement together to an end. But unlike this involvement, "love never ends." It is hoped that your mid-life stresses are more understandable to you now than when we began. But our "knowledge is only a part." The time will come, however, when we "shall understand fully, even as God now understands us fully." Until then we have the spiritual resources for coping, namely, "faith, hope, and love . . .; but the greatest of these is love" (I Cor. 13:12–13).

Suggested Readings

Gray, Madeline. *The Changing Years: The Menopause Without Fear.* Doubleday & Co., 1967.

Howe, Reuel L. *The Creative Years.* Seabury Press, 1959.

Hulme, William E. *Let the Spirit In.* Abingdon Press, 1979.

Mayer, Nancy. *The Male Mid-Life Crisis.* Doubleday & Co., 1979.

O'Neill, Nena and George. *Shifting Gears.* Avon Books, 1975.

Slater, Philip. *The Pursuit of Loneliness: American Culture at the Breaking Point,* rev. ed. Beacon Press, 1976.